Cancer

Experiments and Concepts

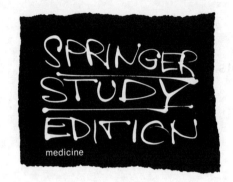

Cancer
Experiments and Concepts

R. Süss

V. Kinzel

J. D. Scribner

Translated from the German
by
J. D. Scribner

Springer-Verlag New York · Heidelberg · Berlin
1973

R. Süss
Senior Research Associate, Experimental Pathology
German Cancer Research Center
Heidelberg, Germany

V. Kinzel
Research Associate, Experimental Pathology
German Cancer Research Center
Heidelberg, Germany

J. D. Scribner
Project Leader, Chemical Carcinogenesis
Pacific Northwest Research Foundation
Seattle, Washington

H. E. Baader
Artist
German Cancer Research Center
Heidelberg, Germany

SPRINGER
STUDY.
EDITION   Design: Peter Klemke, Berlin.

© 1973 by Springer-Verlag New York Inc.

Library of Congress Catalog Card Number 70-189962

Printed in the United States of America.

ISBN 0-387-90042-X Springer-Verlag New York·Heidelberg·Berlin
ISBN 3-540-90042-X Springer-Verlag Berlin·Heidelberg·New York

FOREWORD

This book really ought to be read on vacation, just for enjoyment. Granted, cancer is, literally, a deadly serious matter, and cancer research is primarily a part of medicine with Hippocrates in its background. Yet, cancer research is also natural science, and as such it yields the joys and sorrows of any science. The cancer problem is also a brain teaser, a challenge for the curious.

This introductory report on experimental cancer research is therefore directed to curious students of many disciplines: naturally to medical students, but also to chemists and physicists who have an interest in biological phenomena; biology students will surely encounter problems peculiar to their field in what is supposedly a medical one.

We have attempted to write without assumptions to a certain degree, for a chemist is essentially in over his head in medicine, and a physician has only the slightest idea of the chemical problems important in cancer research. We had no intention of giving a complete view of the field, and from the large number of different lines of development we have chosen only a few. Chemotherapy, as an example, has been treated quite cursorily, along with RNA tumor viruses, although it is possible that just these subjects are especially important for human tumors. Tumor induction via radiation could only be mentioned in passing, in spite of its great practical significance; similarly the role of hormones was only intimated. Impatient readers can without much difficulty delve into single chapters; the more thorough reader will notice that, for this reason, we have not completely avoided repetition.

For those whose knowledge of morphological concepts and tumor nomenclature is lacking, the morphological glossary in the appendix will facilitate understanding of the bulk of the book.

We had no intention of authoring a definitive textbook supplying extensive reference material, for a simple reason. Cancer research has not yet become a graduate degree major in Germany, and is rarely so in the United States (in only one case, as far as the authors are aware). Hence, our purpose is not to give students a monstrous reference book, but to entice those who are completing their studies in the traditional disciplines. We have attempted to refer to original literature by giving the authors' names as often as possible. Further details on any material covered are also available in reviews and other texts of narrower scope.

We thank the following persons for general reading and critical review of single sections: H. Lettré, E. Hecker, D. Schmähl, F. Dallenbach, and K. Goerttler (Heidelberg); H. Friedrich-Freksa, H. Uehleke, and H. Bauer (Tübingen); F. Anders (Giessen) and V. R. Potter (Madison). We are grateful for stimulating discussion with our colleagues G. Kreibich, M. Traut, H. Fischer, F. Marks, and R. Zell, all of whom took the trouble to look through the entire manuscript. We also thank the Verein zur Förderung der Krebsforschung in Deutschland (Prof. K. H. Bauer) for supporting preparation of the illustrations.

Heidelberg, September 1970   R. Süss

V. Kinzel
J. D. Scribner

ABBREVIATIONS AND FREQUENTLY USED CONCEPTS

A	Adenine	G	Guanine
AAF	Acetylaminofluorene	MC	Methylcholanthrene
AB	Aminoazobenzene	NAD	Nicotinamide Adenine
ATP	Adenosine triphosphate		Dinucleotide (formerly
BP	Benzpyrene		DPN)
C	Cytosine	NADH	Hydrogenated from of
D	Total dose		NAD (formerly
d	Daily dose		DPNH)
	(or single dose)	RNA	Ribonucleic acid
DAB	Dimethylaminoazo-	mRNA	messenger RNA
	benzene	S-Phase	Phase in cell cycle in
DBA	Dibenzanthracene		which DNA is
DENA	Diethylnitrosamine		synthesized
DMBA	Dimethylbenz-	SV-40	Simian Vacuolating
	anthracene		Virus
DNA	Deoxyribonucleic acid	T	Thymine

The glossary, which can be consulted directly or via the index, gives information on morphological concepts.

Antibody	A specific protective protein that develops in response to an antigen
Anticarcinogenic	Inhibitory to cancer induction
Antigen	Specific foreign agent capable of eliciting an immune response
Carcinogenic	Induces cancer
Carcinogenesis	The induction of cancer

Cocarcinogenic	Aiding cancer induction. See tumor promotion — development of latent tumor cells. See pp. 53—63.
Cytopathic	Injurious to cells
Lysis	Breakup of a cell, possibly by external damage or virus infection
Lytic, cytolytic	Leading to lysis
Neoplasm	"New growth"; applies to both benign and malignant tumors
Neoplastic transformation	Process leading to conversion of a normal cell into a tumor cell
Oncogenic	Carcinogenic; used to refer to viruses which cause cancer, as "oncogenic viruses"
Syncarcinogenic	Describing the working together of carcinogenic stimuli
Toxic	Crudely, "poisonous" — in contrast to "specific" carcinogenic effects; *cytotoxic* — leading to cell injury and death

CANCER RESEARCH AS NATURAL SCIENCE

Experimental cancer research is a modern interdisciplinary science par excellence: pathologists, biochemists, radiation physicists, virologists, toxicologists, and natural products chemists are working in common to find out what a tumor cell is, how it originates, and how to combat it. Alongside the classifications of the diagnostic pathologist we now find the theoretical models of the molecular biologist; sophisticated biochemical treatments now supplement scalpel and X-ray. The need for interdisciplinary communication in cancer research is evident, yet we are still to a large extent in need of a common language.

Until now medical wishes and hopes have been predominant, and naturally the prevention and combating of cancerous diseases will continue to be the most important stimulus to experimental cancer research. Yet in the last few years there has developed a cancerology, or *oncology*, a biological science of basic research which does not immediately seek practical applications.

Cancer research as a science is not primarily trying to "solve the cancer problem", but wants to approach biological problems from the direction of tumor research. Problems of cell differentiation and growth regulation are the focus of such research, for when one has understood how a tumor cell escapes the normal growth regulation of a higher organism, it is obvious that we will better understand the nature of this regulation itself.

Growth regulation is not the sole object, however; several years ago V. R. Potter characterized the variety of liver tumors with differing degrees of dedifferentiation as a series of "liver mutants", which lend themselves to the study of normal liver function. Normality, paradoxically, is more easily comprehended when it is lacking.

Bacterial genetics learned this a long time ago: bacterial mutants gave the impetus to the development of modern molecular biology. Perhaps in the not too distant future the cancer cell will play a similar role in the development of biology to that already taken by the bacterial cell. Classical molecular biology has come to an end; its "heroic period" (Stent) has run its course; it has reached the point of daring the leap from singlecelled to multicelled organisms, and in this process the distorted picture of the cancer cell may make clear the normal relations between cell and tissue.

Up to now, experimental cancer research has lagged behind general biology; the same old experiments were repeated on tumorous material, and modern methods and concepts were simply transcribed into its own systems. The structure of oncology consequently is an extreme case of colorful patchwork; many walls were erected simultaneously, with no one knowing which should be pushed higher. Many disciplines have been working on their own sections, in some cases without even knowing what else was going on. Yet, this unfinished character, this extensive disconnectedness has its own allure for curiosity.

Jesse Greenstein, author of *Biochemistry of Cancer,* once made the pessimistic observation that, "for some odd reason, cancer research has been the graveyard of many a scientific reputation". This may be because cancer research has traditionally represented the ultimate problem, the challenge remaining for someone who has made accomplishments in other fields. Such an attitude has resulted in posing difficult questions ahead of their time, followed by impatience and unsecured announcements of success.

Modern biology has now made new tools available, making it possible to attack old problems anew. Optimists now look forward to seeing cancer research as the melting pot of methods in modern biological research.

EXPERIMENTAL CANCER RESEARCH: BIOLOGY OF GROWTH REGULATION

Prometheus bound suffered daily from having an eagle tear pieces from his liver, yet survived these barbaric operations. There is even a kernel of physiological truth in this myth: if a part of the liver is removed (partial hepatectomy), it grows back within a few days. In the case of rats the operation is even successful if more than two-thirds of the liver are removed, and it can be performed several times on the same animal. Each time the liver regenerates to its previous size. Each time, however, the regeneration comes to a halt, "invisible boundaries" stop growth, or, as the German proverb puts it, here too, trees do not grow up to the heavens.

Erythrocytes have a lifetime of only 120 days (in man); within this period the entire population of red blood cells is replaced once. For a blood volume of 4 to 6 liters, with 5×10^6 erythrocytes per mm³, this means the production of 6 to 9×10^{13} red blood cells within a single year. Exactly this many cells must be destroyed within the same period, for the total number (disregarding minor variations) remains constant.

Or consider the example of the skin: within 4 to 10 days, all of the cells of mouse epidermis are renewed: more than 1 percent of the cell population of the "basal layer" is constantly in a state of division. Yet in the absence of stimuli, this cell population also remains constant, increase compensated exactly by loss of cells. The constancy of tissue is set as if with a super micrometer.

"Life would like to grow and multiply", once wrote Szent-Györgyi, "but when cells cooperate in the construction of a complex organism, their growth must be regulated in the interest of the whole." A higher organism is possible only by repressive growth politics. These politics must be very rigorous, for a mammalian cell too — not counting exceptions — could double itself every 24 hours. Even the smallest amount of freedom would be fatal: if the production of the epithelial cells which cover the digestive tract were to increase by only a few percent, the system would be completely blocked within a short time. Production and sloughing off therefore must be adjusted to each other in the finest degree.

In a tumor, this adjustment is out of order; a tumor cell no longer reacts to the regulatory impulses of the tissue or the whole organism. It appears to be deaf to growth regulating signals. This is not logically necessary however: a society can be ill, without the necessity of its individual members being so. The individual does not necessarily have to be deaf, if regulatory signals are *drowned out* or *are lacking altogether*. Thus, besides being a problem of individual ethics, cancer appears to be a problem of social ethics — a problem of the rules of community living.

A higher organism is an ecological system in miniature; any changes at any point can influence the entire system. Ecologists can cite examples in which prey "hypertrophies in number" if the predator is eliminated ("population explosion"). In this sense cancer would also be an ecological problem.

Experimental cancer research is therefore always concerned with both: with the tumor cell and the regulatory fields of the organism; it studies the autonomous cancer cell, but must also settle accounts with the host.

TABLE OF CONTENTS

Cancer

Experiments and Concepts

THE IMPETUS FOR EXPERIMENTAL CANCER RESEARCH

Cancer is a "health problem" of the first rank, especially today: in 1900 one in thirty deaths in Germany was due to cancer. Today it is one in five. Only heart disease is a greater killer, and cancer is still on the increase. This staircase in tumor incidence appears to lead further, suggesting that cancer could soon become the most important cause of death.

Naturally we have to be careful with simple mortality statistics: improved diagnosis could lead to an apparent increase in the inci-

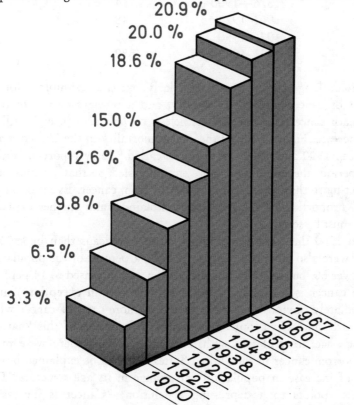

CANCER STAIRCASE: INCREASE IN CANCER MORTALITY

Figure 1

dence of cancer. Then, too, many cases today are probably diagnosed as cancer which earlier would simply have been filed under "old age". Mistakes in diagnosis in either direction are largely excluded from the autopsy rooms of pathology departments, but even here there is impressive evidence that cancer is becoming more frequent. The following table gives the number of cases of lung cancer diagnosed in the Heidelberg Pathology Department for the periods indicated.

Period	Number of Cases
1841–1875	2
1876—1900	14
1901–1925	48
1926–1950	289
1951–1963	589

Granted, lung cancer is a particularly extreme example. Not all forms of cancer increase as rapidly, and a few are even retreating (stomach cancer, for one). Nonetheless, on balance cancer is still on the increase. Figure 2 shows the cancer mortality in the United States between 1900 and 1960 (from the so-called "Terry report"). Within this period, the population more than doubled, so that we must also expect more than twice as many deaths from cancer. Even so, only a small proportion of the increase is explained, and further explanations must be sought.

In 1960 there were not simply more Americans than in 1900 — there were also more old people. In 1900, 7 percent of the population was over 60, but by 1950 this proportion had increased to 14 percent. Since cancer is a disease of old age (with certain exceptions), it is immediately obvious that there should be more cases of cancer when there are more old people. But even with inclusion of this "natural factor", we are still left with a deficit: in 1960, there were more deaths from cancer in the United States than can be explained on the basis of increase in population and change in its age structure. This "excess" points to a depressing conclusion: "Cancer is increasing simply because those things which cause it are increasing" (K. H. Bauer).

This book is concerned in large part with these causes, with a predominant word from experimental cancer research, which has succeeded to date in identifying a whole series of these causes. But

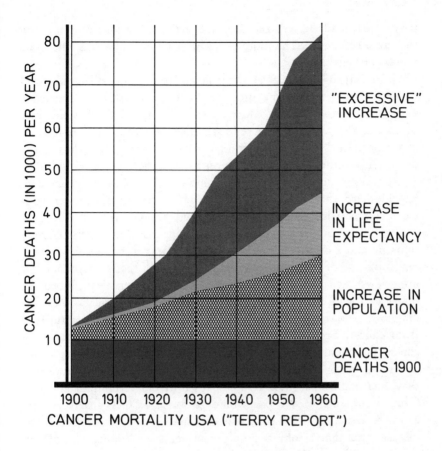

Figure 2

in almost every case, the first clues came from experience with the human disease. Hence we should first scan through clinical experience in order to obtain a clue to the riddle of why more and more people are becoming victims of cancer.

Melancholia Carcinogenica

Melancholy women have a tendency toward cancer, Galen taught, and this was a plausible explanation for him. Hippocrates and Galen too saw a balanced state of health in the well-tempered mixing of the four body humors (blood, phlegm, yellow and black bile). Unbalance meant sickness, and too much black bile (Gr. melas chole) was

3

particularly bad. It was the cause of the more serious diseases, and the cause of cancer. The more pungent this black bile was, the more vile was its effect.

Jean Astruc (1684–1766), a physician from Montpellier, subjected Galen's theory to experimental test 1600 years later: he burned a piece of a breast cancer along with a "normal" beef steak and compared the tastes of the residual ashes. He could not determine any especially "pungent" taste in the cancer ashes, and thus wrote off the "melancholy theory" of cancer as far as he was concerned.

It was by no means forgotten, however; in 1844 it occurred to Rigoni Stern that, among married women, cancer of the cervix is more common in sensitive and frustrated persons. And in 1964, D. M. Kissen wrote that "the evidence suggests that both cigarette smoking and a characteristic personality appear to be involved in the development of cancer." He had conducted many psychological interviews with about 900 patients with chest complaints. When the interviews were held, neither he nor the respective patients knew the diagnosis. It later turned out about half of these patients suffered from cancer. From this comparison between lung cancer and non-cancer pulmonary patients, Kissen characterized the cancer patients as having "poor outlets for emotional discharge". Others wrote that they had confirmed these results with different techniques and different terminologies. No one would go so far as to say that a "lung cancer personality" is a sufficient explanation for occurrence of the disease, and that smoking simply represents an "indicator" of this special psychic constitution — no one, that is, except representatives of the tobacco industry. Still, psycho-physical interactions are again under discussion. Even animal experiments fit into the picture: the Pavlov school has reported that dogs subjected to prolonged experimental neurosis developed spontaneous cancers of the internal organs.

In this connection one might consider investigations conducted by Berkson: according to him, married, single, and divorced men have differing, increasing risks of dying from lung cancer; divorced men die almost twice as often as married men, while the singles lie in between.

All in all, the "melancholia carcinogenica" has not been forgotten. However, it has remained difficult to assess the importance of psychosomatic factors. There is much less discussion about the importance of chemical substances for tumor development in humans. The case most often discussed is cigarette smoking and cancer.

Cigarette Smoking and Lung Cancer

"It is definitely no exaggeration to say that the lung cancer of today is the greatest cancer experiment ever carried out in the history of mankind" (K. H. Bauer). Some pertinent data show why: more than one million U.S. veterans were under observation for more than eight years. It turned out that the number of deaths from lung cancer was ten times higher among smokers than among nonsmokers. The heavy smokers were even worse off: smoking two packs a day or more gave a 24-fold higher risk than that for nonsmokers (Kahn). An English study gave similar results: those who smoked 25 cigarettes or more per day died 20 times more often from lung cancer than did nonsmokers (Doll and Hill).

These and many other data led one epidemiologist to say: "Only the ignorant or prejudiced now deny the reality of the association between cigarette smoking and the incidence of lung cancer" (Fletcher). There are some puzzling facts however.

Cats and dogs are also reported to suffer increasingly from lung cancer. Continuously worsening air pollution seems to be the most obvious candidate for the agent of this increase. If air pollution has something to do with lung cancer, one would expect lung cancer mortality to be higher in cities than in the surrounding open country. And indeed, according to American, English, and Swedish statistics, lung tumor incidence is 2 to 3 times higher in cities than in the country.

Our Daily Carcinogens

Our whole environment is contaminated with cancer-producing substances. We touch them, eat them, and breathe them. It used to be that only certain narrowly circumscribed occupational groups came in contact with carcinogenic substances:
- the English chimney sweep boys (soot from narrow chimneys)
- aniline dye workers (naphthylamine in the early dye factories)
- miners in copper and uranium mines (radiation damage, as well as carcinogenesis by certain metal dusts)
- asbestos workers.

Now, carcinogenic agents have become a worldwide risk for the general population. It is no longer necessary to climb around in narrow chimneys to come into contact with carcinogenic hydrocarbons. 3,4-Benzpyrene, a well-known representative of this class, is found in the air of large cities in concentrations as high as 400 µg/1000 cubic yards. It is constantly being replenished from chimneys and exhaust pipes.

It follows that benzpyrene ought to show up in our food: levels as high as 25 µg/kg have been found in vegetables. Cooking fats and oils have been found to contain 5 to 20 µg/kg. It is not really surprising to run across benzpyrene in smoked foods or even in steaks. Lijinsky and Shubik found between 5 and 50 µg/kg in the outer surfaces of charcoal-broiled steaks. They concluded that polycyclic hydrocarbons are produced by pyrolysis of the fat dripping onto the hot coals. This explains why no benzpyrene could be detected in oven-broiled steaks. This small example also illustrates the problem of cost/benefit ratio, a problem which confronts any producer of food additives, pesticides, or drugs. The American suburbanite can choose to avoid benzpyrene in his steaks and sacrifice the unique flavor obtained from the charbroiling process.

New hazards are coming up: We not only eat ready-made carcinogens, but we are possibly able to manufacture them in our body from harmless precursors. This is the message from recent studies on nitrosamines, a class of substances which has fascinated chemists and cancer researchers for more than ten years now.

They are very easily synthesized by simply mixing a secondary amine with nitrous acid under acidic conditions (nitrous acid is the acid form of nitrite salts).

$$\begin{array}{c}R\\\diagdown\\R\diagup\end{array}NH + HNO_2 \xrightarrow{\ acid\ } \begin{array}{c}R\\\diagdown\\R\diagup\end{array}N{-}NO + H_2O$$

In the simplest case, by reacting dimethylamine with HNO_2 one obtains dimethylnitrosamine, a yellowish liquid with an aromatic odour. The chemical industry considered using it as a solvent, but they reconsidered their plans when it turned out that this substance was toxic for the liver and that it even produced liver cancer (Magee).

This mobilized cancer researchers: A whole series of nitrosamines was synthesized and tested for carcinogenic activity. It turned out that many of these compounds were as powerful carcinogens as simple dimethylnitrosamine. Some of them attacked organs and tissues rarely or never before attacked by other carcinogens. This puzzling versatility was one of the main reasons why very thorough studies were made with these new carcinogens (Druckrey, Preussmann). However, it was not the only one. Field studies were initiated to find out if these substances are part of our chemical environment. This would be no surprise, because some nitrosamines are still used as intermediates in chemical industry (e. g. dimethylnitrosamine is used to prepare dimethylhydrazine, a constituent of rocket fuel).

Quite fortunately, preliminary results indicate that nitrosamines are present in our food only in rather low concentrations. But lately the nitrosamines returned to the scene and opened up rather chilling perspectives.

Since nitrosamines are so easily synthesized in the chemist's test tube, people began to ask whether they can be as easily formed in an animal. Since acid is an important requirement when nitrosamines are formed from amines and nitrile, an animal's stomach would provide a perfect reaction vessel. After first unsuccessful trials it was possible to induce tumors by feeding amines together with nitrite (Sander, also Greenblatt, Mirvish).

This opens up the possibility that by eating "harmless" nitrites (abundant in sausage and certain preserved meat) together with secondary amines which may occur in our food, we might indeed synthesize appreciable amounts of carcinogens ourselves. (Also, transformation of nitrates into nitrites is possible by certain bacteria which occur in our intestinal flora). Special attention has been drawn to certain drugs which contain amines which could be converted into nitrosamines — a sobering example is piperazine which is used in treating worms.

The chemist can accurately predict how easily a nitrosamine is synthesized from its precursors (Mirvish), but cannot tell *a priori* how dangerous a given combination may be for an animal. Rush programs are therefore just being started to find out how great the danger really is.

The Turkey Disaster and the Aflatoxin Story

In 1960, over 100,000 turkey poults died in England from acute hepatic necrosis. This "turkey X" disease was rapidly traced to certain dietary sources: moldy peanut meal had been imported from Brazil and Africa. The poisonous mold was identified as *Aspergillus flavus,* and the toxins produced by this mold were soon isolated and purified and called aflatoxins. These compounds are very poisonous (1 mg/kg can kill a dog, a young rat, or a turkey).

These aflatoxins were not merely poisonous, however: when the rotten peanut meal was fed to rats, the rats developed hepatomas (liver cancer). People would not normally eat moldy peanut meal, but *Aspergillus flavus* can grow in many foods. Aflatoxins have occasionally been found in moldy whole wheat bread, moldy flour and potatoes, and even in wine. It is comforting to know that soft cheeses which have molds (Camembert, Roquefort, Gorgonzola) need not be suspected. Apparently the mold cultures which are added during the cheese production *(Penicillium roqueforti*, for example) suppress foreign infection by the dangerous *Aspergillus flavus*.

Aflatoxins are possibly also responsible for the high incidence of primary liver carcinomas in certain parts of Africa. Suspicion has previously been directed against the protein-deficient diet of the indigenous population, or against certain alkaloids in plants of the *Senecio* family. But occasionally corn supplies in the damp tropic climate are infested with *Aspergillus flavus*.

In the United States and in Europe, rotted food should not be expected to be a cause of cancer. Ironically, however, the measures taken to protect our food supplies have conjured up new carcinogenic risks. Thioacetamide, for example, was introduced as a fungicide; it induces liver cancer in rats. The danger due to insecticides is a particularly grotesque example.

Pesticides or Humanicides

Pesticides have long since stopped causing injury only to pests. Surely DDT can be considered to be in the class of insecticides that are out of control. It has spread over the entire world, it is concentrated in food chains such as plankton-fish-man, and, most unsettling, it is stored for long periods in body fat. Each new dose of DDT is piled on top of what is already there. G. R. Taylor has written sarcastically: "Americans are not fit for human consumption, since they average over 10 ppm of DDT in their body fat, double the amount permitted in food by pure food laws. Nor is American mothers' milk free to cross state lines (except of course in the original container) for similar reasons."

DDT is not strongly active in animal tests, but is definitely accepted as a carcinogen. Let us conclude this short collection of examples from our environmental infestation list with a look at a newcomer.

Asbestos Lung Cancer

Asbestos has become an important raw material in modern technology. Because of its insulating properties, it is used in electrical insulation, in flooring, and in the manufacture of brake linings and transmissions for automobiles. In major construction it is applied to unfinished outer surfaces by high pressure sprays. World consumption has increased from 30,000 tons to 4 million tons in the last 60 years.

Asbestosis in the men who work with this material has been known for a long time: X-rays show characteristic changes in the diseased lungs. Asbestosis has long been recognized as an occupational disease, but it is not the only product of such continued exposure. Doll in England could show that men who had worked in asbestos production for more than 20 years suffered from lung cancer 11 times more frequently than the general population.

Blue Cape asbestos causes a particular type of cancer, previously rare, the so-called mesothelioma, in which the pleura and peritoneum are attacked. "Asbestos bodies" are often found in the lungs of asbestos workers, the result of encapsulation of the asbestos fibers by a yellow-brown substance. But mesotheliomas and asbestos bodies are now being found in patients that had not worked with asbestos.

Is asbestos cancer to become more general than simply an occupational disease? It is hard to guess how great the danger to the general population has become, but just the number of brake linings constantly being worn away is probably a considerable contribution to the problem. J. G. Thompson, an expert on the asbestos problem, predicted that asbestos lung cancer could overtake cigarette lung cancer very soon.

"Morality" and Genital Cancer

American Negro women have a higher rate of genital cancer (cervical carcinoma) than white American women. A study in New York showed this quite clearly (incidence per 100,000 population):

Jewish women	4.7
Other white women	17.1
Negro women	53.6
Puerto Rican women	109.8

Racial differences appear to be responsible for these differences, but stastistics can be deceiving. Investigations in a hospital for the poor in Louisville, Kentucky showed no differences between black and white. Instead it appeared that social standing could explain the cervical carcinoma rates, in this case low social status, coincident with early sexual relations, early age at marriage, and frequent births. This interpretation makes it understandable why women in India often suffer from cervical carcinoma: great poverty is associated with sexual activity very early in their youth.

But let's get back to the above table. Jewish women in New York have a pronouncedly lower tumor incidence than even other white women; correspondingly, Israel reports the lowest incidence of cervical carcinoma in the world. Cancer epidemiologists ascribed this at first to the Jewish custom of circumcision, which results in a lack of accumulation of smegma (a secretion of the penis). Today an examination of the Talmudic rules governing sexual life reveals a whole collection of hygienic prescriptions which could act to prevent cancer.

Not only Jewesses are separate from the remainder of the statistics. Nuns also have a very low chance of suffering from genital cancer. This does not mean that nuns have a lower risk overall. Quite the contrary.

Nuns have an Increased Risk of Breast Cancer

As long as 200 years ago, Ramazzani noticed that in Padua there were more cases of breast cancer among nuns than among married women. This observation was later statistically substantiated.

The risks of breast cancer and genital cancer run counter to each other: breast cancer patients married later and had fewer children than did control patients. The exact opposite was the case for genital cancer. The dependencies on social status also ran counter to each other: breast cancer is more frequent in well-to-do circles, probably simply because marriages take place later and fewer children are born.

Stomach Cancer in the Poor

The remarkable connection between money and cancer is also apparent for stomach cancer:

Social Class	Gastric Cancer Mortality Ratio
Professionals and well-to-do artisans	60
Skilled artisans	100
Laborers and unskilled workers	130

The deeper reason could be deficient diet resulting from relative poverty, but differing dietary habits may also play a role. Weissburger suggested (as an example) that over-salted food could be a contributing factor in the development of stomach cancer.

Until now, cancer of the digestive tract has been especially frequent, and in Germany stomach cancer is still the leading form of cancer. But the proportion of stomach cancer is regressing significantly in many countries. Japan is an important exception. Not only are Japanese much more subject to stomach cancer (5 times more than white Americans): until recently, stomach cancer has *not* regressed in that country. It could be a racial factor, but emigrated Japanese puncture holes in this idea: Japanese-Americans have a much lower incidence than Japanese who remained in their homeland.

The Cancer Staircase Again

Optimists could suppose that the proportion of deaths due to cancer out of the total death rate will not climb as rapidly in the future as in the first half of this century: after all, the upward staircase (p. 1) is clearly flattening out. But the conclusion that carcinogenic influences are on the wane would be in error.

It will be necessary to include in the calculations slowly, ever increasingly noticeable cure rates. Even 50 years ago, the statistics for deaths due to cancer meant the same as statistics for total cancer cases. Today, however, one must clearly distinguish between mortality (proportion of deaths due to cancer) and morbidity (proportion of cases of cancer). This distinction is due to the occasionally amazing therapeutic results, which have been made possible primarily by improved methods for early detection: through early enough recognition of breast cancer, three out of four women can be completely cured of it today.

Nowadays it appears to be not at all unrealistic that carcinoma of the cervix could become a forgotten disease, if the preliminary stages of this form of cancer are recognized soon enough (see page 70).

Summary and Prognosis

Even dinosaurs and the ancient Egyptians had cancer, but it is only in this century that cancer has come close to being the major cause of death. A goodly portion of this dramatic increase lies in the fact that we now have a longer average life span, and that cancer takes its time.

But there are not simply more old people. We also live more dangerously. Our environment is infested with carcinogens. We are even helping to infest it more. Statistical research is elucidating relationships between environment and cancer (smoking and lung cancer; radiation and leukemia; etc.).

It is not always easy for experimental tumor research to relate to these problems. Sure, we can get mice to breathe cigarette smoke, but since the filtering system in their nasal regions differs from that of man, the results obtained can hardly be extrapolated to man.

It is difficult for experimental cancer research to get away from using its standard organs — liver and skin. But liver cancer plays hardly any role in human medicine, and a case of primary hepatoma still causes some excitement among hospital pathologists. Skin cancer is indeed more frequent, but its high cure rate makes it uninteresting for the clinician.

But experimental oncologists must make do with what they have: skin is easy to work with and to observe, and liver offers a wealth of biochemical data. Thus, cancer research without liver and skin is unthinkable, and much important basic knowledge has been obtained from these two "simple" organs. As a result, experimental tumor research has quite naturally gotten somewhat removed from the priority lists of human medicine, but this is hardly a reason to want to be hard on it.

A FIRST STEP: ELUCIDATION OF TAR CANCER

It is probably a doubtful task in many cases to establish the beginning of a science. There are difficulties even for experimental cancer research, yet the year 1775 seems to have particular significance. In that year a French physician, Bernard Peyrilhe, inoculated dogs with human tumors and thereby induced new "growths". The Academie des Sciences et Beaux Arts at Lyon awarded him first prize in a contest which they had established for investigations into the "causes of the cancer virus". Yet both the good doctor and the academy had made a mistake: the growths were not really tumors, but merely pus-containing abscesses; but without microscope and bacteriological techniques, inflammatory swellings and malignant tumors could not be easily distinguished.

In the same year an English physician, Percival Pott, published a report on scrotal cancer in chimney sweeps. These patients had been forced as children to climb around in the narrow English chimneys, to scrape the soot from the inside. Pott realized that he was dealing with malignant tumors, and consequently was the first to diagnose an occupational cancer. Furthermore, he had established the protocol for an *ad hoc* experiment proving that cancer can be evoked by external influences. The "causative agent" in this case was obviously the soot, that is, extremely small coal dust particles adhering together by a tar.

One hundred years after Pott, the German physician Volkmann recognized the tar itself as a cancer-stimulating principle. His proof was in the form of tar workers who developed cancer primarily on their hands and forearms. But not until 140 years after Pott did anyone succeed in inducing cancer in animals: in 1915 the Japanese workers Yamagiwa and Ichikawa reported that they had induced real tumors by painting tar on the ears of rabbits. The critical and envious would only admit to a further confirmation of an already well-known fact; in reality, however, the two Japanese had made a first step in experimental tumor research.

Experimental Tumor Research before Yamagiwa

Granted, it had already been learned how to transplant spontaneous tumors into appropriate receptor animals, and people had begun to investigate the properties and behavior of these "artificial" tumors. Some of those first inoculated tumors, such as the Jensen sarcoma, are still test objects in many cancer research institutes. Basically, however, these tumors were and are nothing but spontaneous tumors which appeared uncontrolledly in an animal, and which, instead of simply on the animal of origin, continued to grow on as many animals as desired. In other words, these were living, permanent preparations from a pathological museum display rather than representative examples for tumorous growth. Most assuredly, however, they were useless for answering the question of how tumors appear to begin with.

The solution of just this question, however, naturally occupied many pathologists of the waning nineteenth century. These attempts at a solution stand out above all the others:

1) Virchow ("Die krankhaften Geschwülste," 1863) maintained that, in the final analysis, cancer is caused by irritation, and he referred expressly to the cases which Pott had analyzed.

2) Cohnheim and Ribbert postulated that fragmented embryonic tissue was to be considered as the starting point for malignant tumors.

3) Finally, many considered the possibility that parasitic organisms induce tumors.

Folke Henschen, a Swedish pathologist and an active eyewitness of these attempts, depicted the climate in a Yamagiwa Memorial Address: "The great progress in microbiology at the end of the 19th century led a series of scientists to seek the cause of all types of cancer in infections with bacteria, fungi, algae, and protozoa, or in infestation with animal parasites of different nature ... I remember clearly when the aged French scientist Borrel took me aside in Paris, hoping to convince me of the significance of Ascarides as carcinogenic factors ... The original parasite hypotheses were soon abandoned but they revived anew, as we know, in the viral hypothesis." The resurrection came quickly: in 1908 and 1910 the first viral tumors were discovered, but official cancer research took no notice.

At the turn of the century, the Cohnheim-Ribbert hypothesis was especially in vogue: "I heard pathologists speaking a little arrogantly about Virchow's 'old' irritation theory as belonging to the past."

Virchow's irritation theory was nevertheless the stimulus for uncounted attempts to induce cancer experimentally via "external irritants," yet all these attempts were unsuccessful. "All these negative experiments caused an atmosphere of resignation in many quarters," Henschen summarized. "Cancer seemed to remain something inaccessible."

Under these conditions one can imagine how relieved the pathologists were, when Yamagiwa and Ichikawa reported in 1915 on their "Experimental Studies on Atypical Epithelial Proliferation."

Yamagiwa and Ichikawa Induce the First Experimental Tumors

The two Japanese used a very simple method: 2 to 3 times a week they applied tar to the inside of rabbits' ears with a glass rod. After only 3 months wartlike proliferations developed at the site of application; later larger growths were formed which eventually more or less turned entire ears into cancerous growths.

"Fortune and fortitude" played equal parts: only continuous painting over months permitted the induction of papillomas and carcinomas. If they had used dogs or guinea pigs, however, even inhuman patience would not have brought results.

It was quickly learned that simple painting of tar preparations on the backs of mice could also lead to the production of benign and malignant tumors. This was a considerable simplification: these smaller animals could be kept easier than rabbits, permitting the usage of much larger numbers of animals. Then too, the time required to wait for tumors was considerably shorter. Consequently, mice became standard animals for experimental cancer research, so much so that the National Cancer Institute was occasionally jokingly referred to as the "National Mouse Institute."

The next question was obvious: which substances in tar were the actual inducers of the papillomas and carcinomas? In spite of the "convenient" mice, the answer seemed unattainable, for tar chemistry was still in its infancy, and little more was known other than the fact that tar is a mixture of many different substances. Unfortunately, this was not the only difficulty; in order to test partially purified tar fractions for their carcinogenic properties, it was necessary to wait months to find out if such-and-such a fraction was active or inactive. It is clear that multistep purification processes, which are the rule for complicated mixtures, must in themselves be tremendously time-consuming.

A Few Grams of 3,4-Benzpyrene from Two Tons of Tar

In spite of all this, Cook, Hewitt, and Hieger attempted the isolation of a pure carcinogen from coal tar. Besides patience these English scientists also possessed courage: they did not rely at all on biological tests that would have required months of waiting; rather, they used a physicochemical characteristic. It had already been noticed that all tars tested at that time displayed the same fluorescence spectrum. This "signal" appeared even more valuable when it was realized that a pure compound, 1,2-benzanthracene, showed almost the same spectrum. Therefore, they had confidence that they could isolate a pure compound; with a little luck, it might also be a carcinogen.

Cook had two tons of tar fractionally distilled at the municipal gas works. After multiple further distillations, crystallizations, and the preparation of characteristic derivatives these men succeeded in isolating 50 grams (2.5×10^{-6} percent yield!) of an as yet unknown substance. The new compound was 3,4-benzpyrene, and was shown to be a useful carcinogen by biological testing.

3,4-Benzpyrene was certainly not the very first pure carcinogen. In 1929, Cook had already synthesized 1,2,5,6-dibenzanthracene (DBA), which also proved to be a good carcinogen.

3,4-Benzpyrene and 1,2,5,6-DBA belong to the class of polycyclic hydrocarbons. Members of this group are derived from the basic building block benzene, which can be combined in manymembered ring systems with numerous variations (Figure 3).

Polycyclic Hydrocarbons can Induce Tumors other than Skin Tumors

A single subcutaneous injection of 7,12-dimethylbenzanthracene (DMBA), 3,4-benzpyrene (BP), or of other carcinogenic hydrocarbons leads to sarcomas after a somewhat long latent period (3 to 4 months, depending on dosage). In this test rats are considerably more sensitive than mice.

If DMBA is injected subcutaneously into newborn mice, multiple lymphomas occur (lymph gland tumors), and the usual sarcomas at the injection site are seldom found. Ovarian tumors appear in mice if DMBA is fed, injected intraperitoneally, or simply painted on the back. Rats on the other hand respond with mammary carcinomas. In

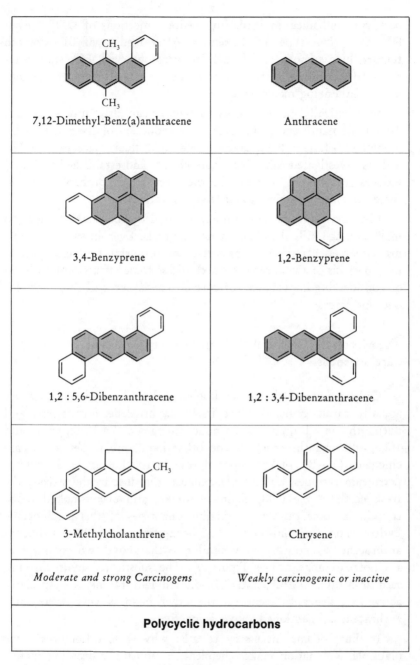

7,12-Dimethyl-Benz(a)anthracene	Anthracene
3,4-Benzyprene	1,2-Benzyprene
1,2 : 5,6-Dibenzanthracene	1,2 : 3,4-Dibenzanthracene
3-Methylcholanthrene	Chrysene
Moderate and strong Carcinogens	*Weakly carcinogenic or inactive*

Polycyclic hydrocarbons

Figure 3

both rats and mice, multiple intravenous injections of DMBA even lead to various types of leukemias. After feeding of BP, stomach tumors, lung tumors, and leukemias were observed. Hamsters react to DMBA painting with malignant melanomas (tumors of the pigment-synthesizing melanocytes).

Paradoxically, polycyclic hydrocarbons can also suppress cancer: 3-methylcholanthrene (MC) blocks the induction of liver tumors by 3'-methyl-4-dimethylaminoazobenzene and 2-fluorenylacetamide. The Millers investigated this effect more closely and established that MC induces microsomal enzymes in the liver which probably convert these carcinogenic amines to inactive derivatives.

Like most carcinogens, polycyclic hydrocarbons are toxic: too high a dosage kills the experimental animals. Even in surviving animals toxic effects are often apparent (necrotic skin on local application, necrosis of the adrenal cortex). These toxic effects could also be of considerable importance for carcinogenesis: we will return to this question later.

Theories on the Chemical Mechanism of Hydrocarbon Carcinogenesis

Only a few of the many known polycyclic hydrocarbons are actually carcinogenic. Benzene itself, naphthalene, anthracene, and phenanthrene all appear to be noncarcinogenic. 3,4-Benzpyrene and 1,2,5,6-dibenzanthracene, on the other hand, are rather good carcinogens. (3,4-BP plays a special role in the human environment: petroleum residues, automobile exhaust, the dust in the streets, the fresh earth in the field, cigarette smoke, and even smoked foods contain in some cases nonnegligible quantities of this carcinogenic hydrocarbon.) Astonishingly, 1,2-benzpyrene and 1,2,3,4-dibenzanthracene, structurally very similar to the above two compounds, are not carcinogenic (see Figure 3). The substituted hydrocarbons, such as 3-MC, DMBA, and 9,10-dimethylanthracene are especially active. 1,2-Benzanthracene on the other hand is very weak, and anthracene, as mentioned above, is inactive.

It thus becomes necessary to ask: why these differences? One plausible explanation makes chemical reactivity the deciding factor. Reactive substances would as a consequence be carcinogenic. Additions and substitutions are the basic reaction types to consider; it is addition which has played the greatest role in the history of theoretical explanation of carcinogenic activity. As an example, consider the reaction of polycyclic hydrocarbons with osmium tetroxide:

The mechanism is not known in all its particulars, but as a simplification we can say that a double bond is localized to initiate the reaction. Double bonds which are localized easier than others are often called in these compounds "K-regions." The following table encourages the idea that, in fact, reactivity and carcinogenic activity are parallel: (Table 1).

Table 1: Addition to K-region and Carcinogenic Activity

Hydrocarbon	Rate of OsO_4-Fixation	Carcinogenic Activity
Benzene	0	—
Phenanthrene	0.2	—
1,2-Benzanthracene	1	+
1,2,5,6-Dibenzanthracene	1	+ +
3,4-Benzpyrene	2	+ + +

The limits of this simple comparison are reached quickly: 1,2-benznaphthacene, for example, is very reactive, but not carcinogenic. Still, the basic idea that chemical and carcinogenic activity are related need not be wrong. Certainly, however, the rate of osmium tetroxide fixation reflects only a small portion of an extensive spectrum of chemical reaction possibilities.

In the Pullmans' theory, for example, a significant contribution is said to come from the so-called L-region (with *para*-situated reactive atoms): according to this theory, only the combination of an "active K-region" with an "inactive L-region" permits tumor-inducing properties.

Recently the idea that an epoxide of a carcinogenic hydrocarbon might be a necessary intermediate reactive form has increasingly become an object of study (Sims, Gelboin, Heidelberger). Such epoxides are more effective transforming agents in tissue culture than the parent hydrocarbons, but are not more effective carcinogens in the whole animal. In spite of such difficulties, study of the epoxides appears to be the most promising approach to determining the reactive forms of the hydrocarbons.

Although it is preferable to measure directly the reactivities of the many possible intermediates, this is impractical. Wave mechanical calculations, with paper and pencil or with computers, yield indices which qualitatively indicate relative reactivities among the different hydrocarbons. Calculations of this type are often dignified with the name of "Wave Mechanical Theory of Carcinogenesis." However, in every case we are merely postulating that a certain *type* of reaction is necessary for carcinogenesis, and we try to correlate the calculated susceptibility toward this reaction with carcinogenic activity.

Polycyclic Hydrocarbons are Bound to Protein

Polycyclic hydrocarbons give a strong blue-white to yellow-white fluorescence in ultraviolet light. Using this highly sensitive detection property, E. C. Miller discovered in 1951 that 3,4-benzpyrene is bound to mouse skin protein. These experiments were the out-growth of earlier experiments which succeeded in showing the binding of carcinogenic azo dyes to liver protein (see page 36). Apparently, then, carcinogens bind to proteins of the organs in which they induce tumors.

Heidelberger carried these experiments further using radioactive hydrocarbons. The result was most disappointing: not only carcinogenic, but also noncarcinogenic hydrocarbons were bound to the soluble skin proteins. Thus, the protein-carcinogen reaction seemed to be excluded as a key reaction in carcinogenesis. Then new experiments made "protein-binding" interesting again: Abell and Heidelberger separated the soluble proteins of mouse skin by starch-gel electrophoresis and discovered that the carcinogenic hydrocarbons were preferably bound to a certain slightly basic protein fraction, while noncarcinogenic compounds were smeared over many of the fractions.

Here was signified an important extension of the chemical theory of tumor induction: obviously not only the chemical reactivity of the carcinogen is important, but also the reactivity of the partner, in this case a certain class of protein.

Proteins Could be Growth Regulators

The Millers had already postulated for the azo dyes that binding is not to just any protein, but to growth-regulating proteins. Using this conception, we arrive at a very simple model of a tumor cell: the loss of growth-regulating substances leads automatically to uncontrolled cell divisions. Carcinogens deactivate these regulator proteins, which in turn can no longer be replaced; thus, tumor cells arise in which these proteins are permanently lacking. Twenty years ago this was by no means an unreasonable proposition, for at that time many believed that proteins were responsible for their own reproduction (protein matrix for protein synthesis).

In the interim, however, the prevalent opinion — in fact, dogma — has become that nucleic acids are responsible for the specific structures of protein. Thus, the proteins were dropped to second rank of the cellular hierarchy. Wouldn't carcinogens really have to react with nucleic acids, and with DNA especially?

Polycyclic Hydrocarbons also React with DNA

For a long time the binding of carcinogenic hydrocarbons to DNA of mouse skin remained undemonstrated. The reasons were simple: relatively few molecules are bound, and they can therefore be found only when highly radioactive compounds are used. Even with the use of such "hot" material, extreme care must be used in measuring techniques in order to detect the extremely low radioactivity present.

Brookes and Lawley were the first ones to demonstrate conclusively that polycyclic hydrocarbons are bound to DNA. They found further that binding and carcinogenic activity appeared to be correlated, although Goshman and Heidelberger could not completely reproduce this correlation. The subject of reactions with DNA is the subject of a separate chapter (see page 193), which should be consulted for a more detailed discussion. Meanwhile, let us turn to another class of chemical carcinogens, the aromatic amines.

Summary

Yamagiwa and Ichikawa induced the first experimental tumors with a chemical substance (tar cancer in rabbits, 1915). The primary carcinogenic principles of tar were shown to be polycyclic hydro-carbons, among which are the well-known 3,4-benzpyrene and 3-methylcholanthrene. Not all polycyclic hydrocarbons are carcino-genic; small molecular variations suffice to suppress carcinogenic activity (compare 3,4-benzpyrene and 1,2-benzpyrene).

Attempts have been made to establish a connection between carcinogenic activity and chemical reactivity of these hydrocarbons. Besides chemical reactivity, however, the reactivity of the reaction partner is also important, potential partners being protein, RNA, and DNA.

The active principles in the induction of cancer by tars are known or easily imagined. How these principles work, however, is largely unknown.

AROMATIC AMINES:
ACTIVATION THROUGH METABOLISM

As dye factories, large and small, sprang up in Europe in the last half of the nineteenth century, not only were dyes produced, but also tumors. In the beginning, of course, this danger could not be foreseen. The first aniline dyes had been discovered in England and France, but large-scale production of these dyes followed soon after in Ger-many, too. The name of the huge chemical firm Badische Anilin- und Sodafabrik (BASF) is still a reminder of this first generation of synthetic dyes.

Alfred von Nagel gives a clear picture of the early techniques:

The preparaton of fuchsin took place in a fuchsin melt *via* oxidation of the so-called "Anilinöl für Rot," a mixture of aniline and to-luidines, as then obtained by the production of aniline from in-completely purified benzene. To prepare these melts, a mixture of "Anilinöl für Rot" had to be stirred with an arsenious acid solu-tion in enameled cast-iron kettles above an open fire 6–8 hours at 170–180° C. Unused aniline distilled off and condensed in cooled lead spirals. The fused melts were then dissolved in boiling water in iron digesting pots. On the addition of salt and hydrochloric acid, fuchsin hydrochloride was then formed and allowed to crys-tallize out. In order to cool the solution as slowly as possible and thus obtain the largest possible crystals, the liquid was covered with floating planks, on which the most beautiful crystals formed. Crystallization lasted six weeks, even longer in midsummer. Finally, the cover was removed, the liquid drained off, the crystals collected and set out on racks to dry. The dry crystals were then sorted by hand according to size and beauty, for the quality of the fuchsin was evaluated according to the appearance of the crystals.

Other aniline dyes of constantly expanding palette were later prepared using similarly incautious methods.

Aniline Cancer: Aniline Itself is not to Blame

Even in 1895 the Frankfurt surgeon Rehn was already reporting the increasing appearance of bladder cancer among dye factory workers. In spite of the limited number of patients, Rehn concluded that aniline must have something to do with the occurrence of these tumors. Over the years this suspicion became even stronger, and people began to talk not only about aniline dyes, but also about aniline cancer. Even workers who had long since stopped working in the dye factories (up to 35 years) could still come down with bladder cancer.

To be sure, it finally turned out that aniline itself had not caused these tumors. Instead of aniline, a whole series of other aromatic amines were blacklisted, primarily β-naphthylamine, but also benzidine and diphenylamine. Today careless traffic with these dangerous intermediates is becoming more and more limited, and a few of those products have been completely taken out of production. As an example, the synthesis of free β-naphthylamine has now been bypassed in the production of dyes.

The azo dyes play a special role in the story of the aromatic amines. This new class of dyes had followed the aniline dyes fuchsin and mauve very quickly; it is noteworthy for a wide range of variations in hues and other properties. The carcinogenicity of the azo dyes was again, however, only recognized later, although there were clear warnings early on.

Butter Yellow and the Carcinogenic Azo Dyes

Scarlet Red (also known as Biebrich Scarlet) had very quickly become talked about in medicine (Figure 4). In 1906, Fischer-Wasels

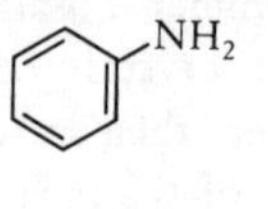

Anilin
(Aminobenzene)

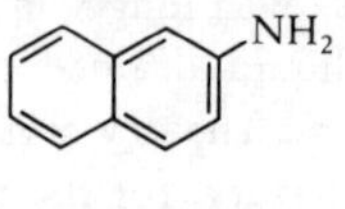

β-Naphthylamine
(2-Aminonaphthalene)

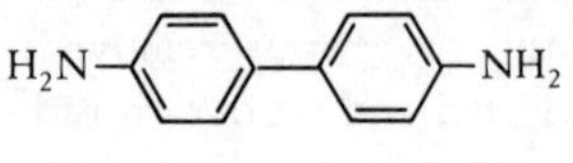

Benzidine

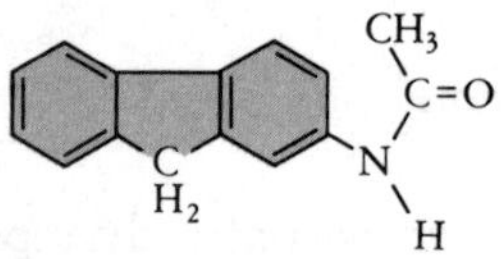

2-Acetylaminofluorene (AAF)

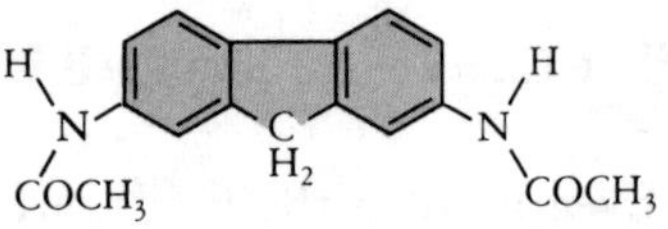

N-N'-2,7-Fluorenylbis-acetamide

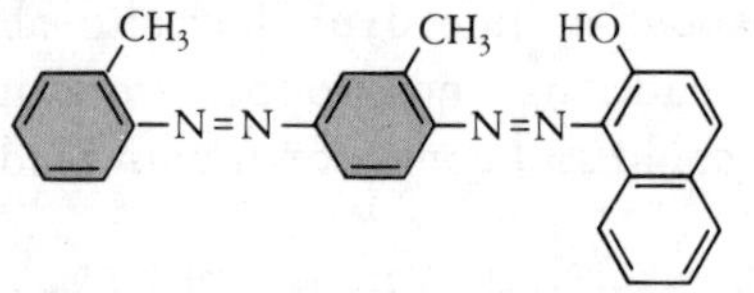

"scarlet-red"

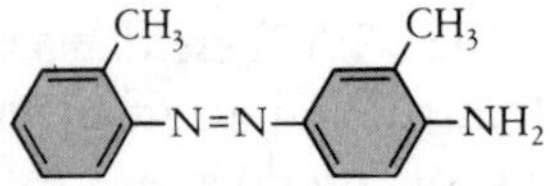

o-Amino-azotoluene

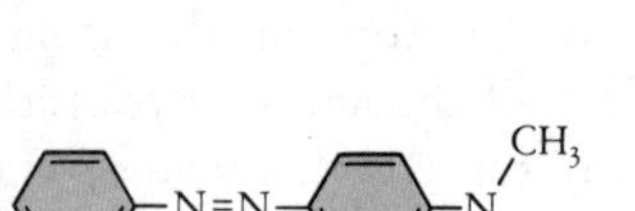

azobenzene (DAB)
("Butter-yellow")

Aromatic amines and azodyes

Figure 4

had noticed epithelial proliferation in the ears of rabbits after he had given multiple subcutaneous injections of a solution of Scarlet Red in oil. People concluded that the dye acted to stimulate growth, and thus it happened that this dye found extensive use in wound therapy to accelerate the regeneration of skin tissue.

It was only after another 30 years that Sazaki and Yoshida discovered the carcinogenic effect of o-aminoazotoluene, a structural component of Scarlet Red. Rats had been given a rice diet containing o-aminoazotoluene in oil. All the rats which survived more than 255 days developed hepatomas. After this discovery, numerous substances, primarily azo dyes, were tested for carcinogenic activity. Soon after (1936), Kinosita identified N,N-dimethyl-4-aminoazobenzene as an even stronger carcinogen than aminoazotoluene. The trivial name for dimethylaminoazobenzene (DAB) is butter yellow, a name derived from the practice (now fortunately given up) of adding this dye to margarine or winter butter to add back the color of summer freshness.

Acetylaminofluorene, an Aborted Insecticide

In 1940, acetylaminofluorene (Figure 4) was patented as the principal ingredient for an insecticide. Before it was put into production, however, it was subjected to thorough testing, including a test for possible carcinogenic activity. By 1941 it was clear that 2-acetylaminofluorene is a highly effective carcinogen. Tumors can be induced in rats, mice, dogs, cats, rabbits, and chickens; bladder and liver tumors are predominant, but mammary tumors, lung tumors, and uterine carcinomas also appear. In most experiments 2-acetylaminofluorene has been added to the diet. It is locally inactive, that is, no tumors are found at the site of injection when this method of administration is used. After all this, the use of 2-acetylaminofluorene as a pesticide was out of the question.

2-Acetylaminofluorene is really an amide (of acetic acid). We will see, however, that it logically is in the same class as the aromatic amines already mentioned. We have now mentioned the most important representatives of these amines: β-naphthylamine, the azo dyes, and aminofluorenes. Let us now consider these substances more closely, in particular, let us become acquainted with their behavior in metabolism.

Not all Aminoazo Dyes are Carcinogenic

By no means are all aminoazo dyes carcinogenic. The basic skeleton, 4-aminoazobenzene (AB), for example, is very weak, if at all active. N-Methyl-4-aminoazobenzene and DAB are strongly active. If the "second" benzene ring is substituted with an extra methyl group in the appropriate position, one obtains the very strong carcinogen, 3'-methyl-N,N-dimethyl-4-aminoazobenzene. If this extra methyl group is located one position away instead (on the opposite end from the amino group), the compound now obtained (4'-methyl-DAB) is almost inactive.

Aminoazo dyes like DAB usually induce only liver tumors. The other aromatic amines are less specific and induce tumors in other organs as well. The example of N,N'-2,7-fluorenyl(bis)acetamide is particularly dramatic; this substance in the rat alone leads to mammary tumors, skin tumors, lung tumors, leukemias, lymphomas, stomach cancer, intestinal tumors, uterine carcinomas, liver tumors, and tumors of the ear duct gland. The frequency of the varied possibilities differs depending on whether administration is by feeding or intraperitoneal injection.

Aromatic Amines Must be Converted to Carcinogens via Metabolism

Aromatic amines as such are noncarcinogenic. Georgiana Bonser was forced to this conclusion from her experiments with β-naphthylamine. She had mixed β-naphthylamine with paraffin, pressed them into small pellets, and implanted them directly into the bladders of her experimental animals. Subsequently, however, only rare tumors appeared, even though feeding of β-naphthylamine induced bladder tumors in dogs, rabbits, and evff guinea pigs.

This experiment showed clearly that at least β-naphthylamine does not act directly to produce tumors. We must assume that somewhere in the organism there is a transformation into an active form. After feeding, the amine passes through numerous organs, with many opportunities to be converted chemically. Thus, it is understandable that β-naphthylamine is carcinogenic on feeding, but inactive on direct implantation into the bladder.

It was quite natural that interest in many laboratories centered on the metabolic products formed in organisms from aromatic amines.

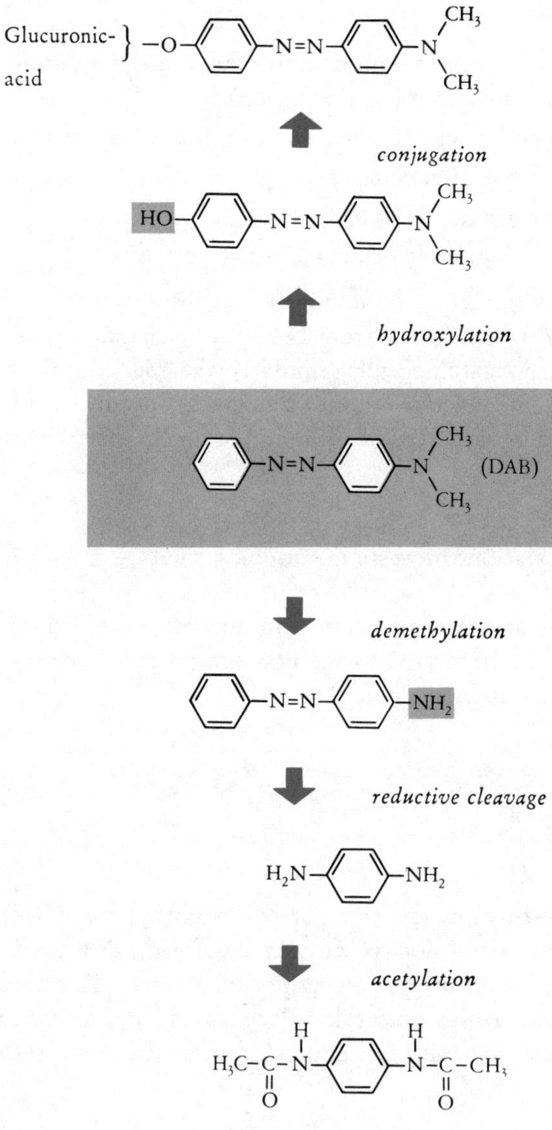

Some metabolites of DAB

Figure 5

The results of the earlier investigations can be quickly summarized (Figure 5):

a) acetylation and deacetylation can take place (addition or removal of an acetyl group at the amino group)

b) azo dyes can be reductively cleaved at the azo group

c) *N*-methyl groups can be removed

d) the aromatic rings can be hydroxylated

e) conjugation with glucuronic acid (see also page 69).

Removal of the methyl group is obviously not the reaction we are looking for. The AB which results from DAB in this manner is, as we have already seen, noncarcinogenic. Similarly the reduction of the azo group results in inactive (noncarcinogenic) products. Only hydroxylation could be suspected of being important in the activation of aromatic amines.

Ortho-ring hydroxylation: Increase in Carcinogenicity

Oxidation of the aromatic ring results in phenols. As an example, β-naphthylamine (I) is converted to the new substance 1-hydroxy-2-aminonaphthalene, an aminophenol.

(I)   (II)

Characteristically — or so people thought — α-naphthylamine (III) is noncarcinogenic: the 1-position is already occupied, this position cannot be oxidized, and so activation cannot take place. Why oxidation at the 2-position, which does take place, should not also be an activation step seems to have been explained away by some rather dubious reasoning.

(III)

The production of phenols from aromatic amines plays a large role, quantitatively. All of the species investigated — rat, mouse, rabbit, dog — excrete considerable quantities of 1-hydroxy-2-amino-naphthalene (II) in the urine on feeding of β-naphthylamine. There are differences, however: the more carcinogenic β-naphthylamine is in a species, the more phenol is excreted by that species. From such comparative metabolism studies, Bonser and Clayson came to the conclusion that the *ortho*-amino phenols represent a step on the path to the actual carcinogen.

Following these indirect indications, Bonser and her coworkers were concerned to test this hypothesis directly. It was easy to raise the criticism that the aminophenols are nothing but detoxification products which are more water soluble than the parent amines and more easily excreted. If ring hydroxylation really were important for the activation of aromatic amines to carcinogens, then the amino-phenols would have to be better carcinogens. One should expect that synthetic aminophenols could induce bladder tumors directly instead of requiring the tortuous path through the body as with β-naphthyl-amine. Therefore, Bonser and her coworkers synthesized a whole series of *ortho*-hydroxy derivatives of the corresponding carcino-genic aromatic amines and tested these derivatives and the parent compounds directly in the bladders of mice. Again, the compounds were mixed with paraffin, formed into pellets, and surgically im-planted.

The results were inconclusive: although β-naphthylamine induced almost no tumors, 1-hydroxy-2-aminonaphthalene was clearly car-cinogenic. Yet, there were other o-hydroxyamines which were not carcinogenic in this test. Several which were active in this test were inactive on feeding.

It is incorrect to say that the *ortho*-hydroxylation hypothesis is false, for there are several aromatic amines that are unquestionably more carcinogenic after ring hydroxylation. On the other hand, this hypothesis does not appear to be generally applicable. More recent work has now discovered a new reaction series that does appear to have this general applicability.

N-hydroxylation, a Necessary but not Always Sufficient Step for Activation of Aromatic Amines

In 1960 Cramer and the Millers reported a new substance isolated from the urine of rats who had been fed 2-acetylaminofluorene

(AAF) for many weeks: this new metabolite differed from AAF by an oxygen attached to the nitrogen, and was called N-hydroxy-2-acetylaminofluorene (N-OH-AAF).

The metabolism of AAF had already been thoroughly studied in great detail by the Weisburgers at the National Cancer Institute in Bethesda. However, they had never followed the excretion products over an extended time. It was just this extra effort which enabled the discovery of N-OH-AAF, since only in the course of time are detectable amounts of this metabolite excreted.

Paper chromatography played a major role in all these investigations. Even the Millers had simply discovered a "new spot" on the paper chromatograms of their urine extracts. Naturally, it is hardly enough to discover a new spot on a paper chromatogram. The spot must be characterized: microanalyses have to be carried out to identify the material giving rise to the spot. Finally, the proposed compound can be synthesized and compared with the product isolated from the rats.

N-OH-AAF was now synthesized in large quantities and fed to rats. It soon turned out that N-OH-AAF is more carcinogenic than AAF: it induces tumors faster and at sites where AAF does not induce tumors. It was shown that N-OH-AAF induces tumors in guinea pigs, even though AAF is noncarcinogenic in these animals. N-Hydroxylation is a general reaction in rats and man. The N-hydroxy derivatives derived from many different carcinogenic amines and amides are more carcinogenic than the non-hydroxylated starting materials. There are no cases in which the N-hydroxylated derivative is less carcinogenic than the parent amine, and several (including α-naphthylamine) in which N-hydroxylation converted noncarcinogenic amines into carcinogens. Still, there remained cases in which N-hydroxylation was ineffective for activation.

In spite of this slight limitation, it appeared more and more that N-hydroxylation represents a necessary step in the activation of carcinogenic aromatic amines; but it might not be entirely sufficient.

The Millers coined the expression "proximate carcinogens" for the *N*-hydroxylated forms of carcinogenic amines, a term describing substances which are more closely related to the actual active forms of the carcinogens than are the parent amines. Research development did not stop at the stage of "proximate carcinogens." From the Miller laboratory came the first indications of how further activated "ultimate carcinogens" could arise from the "proximate" forms. Planned experiments and pure chance contributed equally to this next phase.

Aminoazo Dyes also Form N-hydroxy Derivatives

When attempts were made to apply the *N*-hydroxy story to the azo dyes, it was found to be very difficult to synthesize the corresponding *N*-hydroxy compounds. An elegant method was found, however, for preparing *N*-OH-AB (I) and *N*-OH-acetyl-AB (II).

$$(I) \qquad\qquad (II)$$

(Both of these compounds were then isolated from the urine of rats fed AB.)

There has been no success, however, in attempts to prepare *N*-OH-*N*-methyl-AB (III).

$$(III)$$

Yet it is just this compound which would have been most important, for *N*-methyl-AB (MAB) is carcinogenic, while AB is not. An attempt was then made to approach *N*-OH-MAB by the back door: although (III) could not be synthesized, its ester could be prepared in one step from MAB.

$$(IV)$$

This ester was imagined to be very easily hydrolyzed, and could conceivably yield "transient" free N-OH-MAB. Relatively large quantities were prepared and the testing for carcinogenicity begun.

At this point let us put off discussing the biological results and instead consider another project going on in the Miller group at that time, a project which seemed to have nothing to do with N-hydroxylation.

Azo Dyes React with Methionine

The metabolic products of the azo dyes had been analyzed primarily using column chromatography. In an example analysis, DAB was injected intraperitoneally into a rat, the rat killed after a day, the liver removed and homogenized, digested with cold KOH, and the digestion mixture extracted with a mixture of benzene and hexane. After further purification of the extract, the mixture of dyes was then separated on an alumina column. Unchanged DAB, MAB, and AB were easily separated by this method and demonstrated. Thus the Millers had demonstrated the demethylation of DAB in the rat as early as 1945.

In the late 1950's a new separation method had come into wide use — gas chromatography. In this method, the analysis mixture is vaporized and carried through a separating tube by a carrier gas, such as argon or helium. Depending on the nature of the stationary phase (the packing in the tube), the various substances in the gas are held back to different degrees, thus leading to separation. Gas chromatography is not only a more novel method than paper or column chromatography, but it is also faster and more sensitive and usually gives better separation.

The capability of the gas chromatographic method to separate DAB from its demethylation products was tested as a prelude to other studies on the alkyl groups attached to the nitrogen of AB; the other studies never took place, however, for on the first experiment with a dye mixture obtained from a rat, four peaks were found instead of the three which were expected.

What was the new peak? After it was first shown to really be a dye, small amounts were subjected to microchemical tests to answer preliminary questions. Then hundreds of rats were killed, hundreds of livers homogenized, digested, and extracted, until finally 250 micrograms, a relatively large quantity, was collected as a yellow film on the bottom of a sample bottle. Infrared spectra gave the final clues, and the possible compound was synthesized for comparison. The known and the unknown compounds were the same, 3-methylmer-capto-N-methyl-4-aminoazobenzene (V):

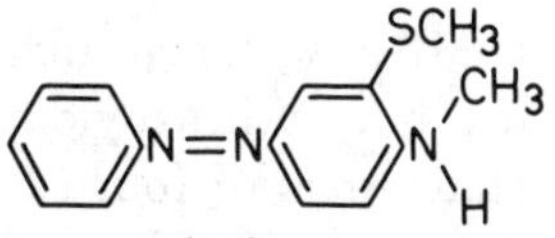

(V)

The obvious logical step was to conclude that the CH₃S-group was derived from methionine. If this were the case, however, then methionine ought to react with MAB. MAB was known to be inactive in this reaction. However, the N-hydroxy derivative seemed a likely possibility, since such derivatives had been found from metabolism of all the other amines studied.

Unfortunately, N-OH-MAB was not available, but its benzoate ester (IV) was in hand. In actual fact, it was enough to simply mix N-benzoyloxy-MAB and methionine, followed by treatment with cold alkali, to obtain 3-CH₃S-MAB.

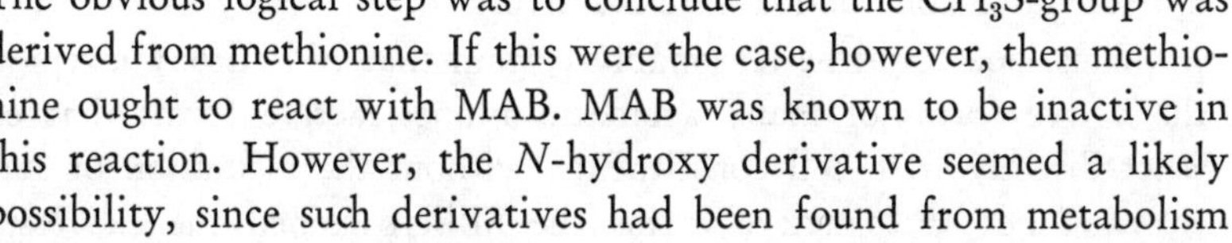

If one waited long enough (4 hours), even the alkali was unnecessary. In no case was an enzyme required for the reaction. Thus, a direct reaction had been brought about between an "activated" carcinogen and a cell component. At this stage there were only two more immediate questions: was it the ester itself which reacted? Was the ester carcinogenic?

N-hydroxy Esters as Final Steps in the Activation to the Actual Carcinogen ("Ultimate Carcinogens")

The first of the above two questions was tested with N-OH-AAF and its ester, N-acetoxy-AAF. Here there was no question: the N-hydroxy derivative, as in previous studies, gave no detectable product with methionine; its acetate ester, however, gave amounts of 3-CH$_3$S-AAF large enough for elementary analysis and other characterization studies. N-Acetoxy-AAF and N-benzoyloxy-MAB were also both found to react with guanosine, a component of RNA.

Finally, the question of carcinogenicity was answered in entirely satisfactory experiments. MAB was noncarcinogenic when injected intramuscularly into rats, but N-benzoyloxy-MAB was a strong carcinogen. Also, the acetate esters of four carcinogenic N-hydroxy-amides (including N-OH-AAF) were all stronger carcinogens by the same test than were the N-hydroxy compounds. Here, too, the non-hydroxylated compounds were inactive.

Thus, one could be reasonably certain that N-hydroxy esters are the active forms of many aromatic amines, active forms that can react directly with cell constituents, without the mediation of some enzyme. For these active forms the Millers coined the expression "ultimate carcinogen."

But which esters are actually formed in the cell? The benzoate esters were obviously out of the question, for benzoic acid is not involved in normal metabolism. Acetate, phosphate, and sulfate were all much better candidates, for all of these ions are in plentiful supply and are found in "activated" forms which facilitate their reactions with appropriate partners (acetyl-CoA as a prime example).

Which Esters are the "Ultimate Carcinogens"?

Besides the easily prepared benzoate and acetate esters, sulfate esters were also prepared. All three esters of N-OH-AAF reacted in vitro with methionine, especially the sulfate. King and Phillips then performed experiments with liver homogenates which seemed to show that both phosphate and sulfate esters are formed, but the Millers could confirm only the formation of sulfates. DeBaun and the Millers then did a detailed study of the "sulfotransferase" system, establishing its existence beyond reasonable doubt and revealing more of its detailed characteristics.

The conversion of an aromatic amide (such as AAF) into its active form thus appears to follow the pathway: amide → N-hydroxy-amide ("proximate carcinogen") → N-sulfate ester ("ultimate carcinogen") (Figure 6). Both the methionine and guanosine binding

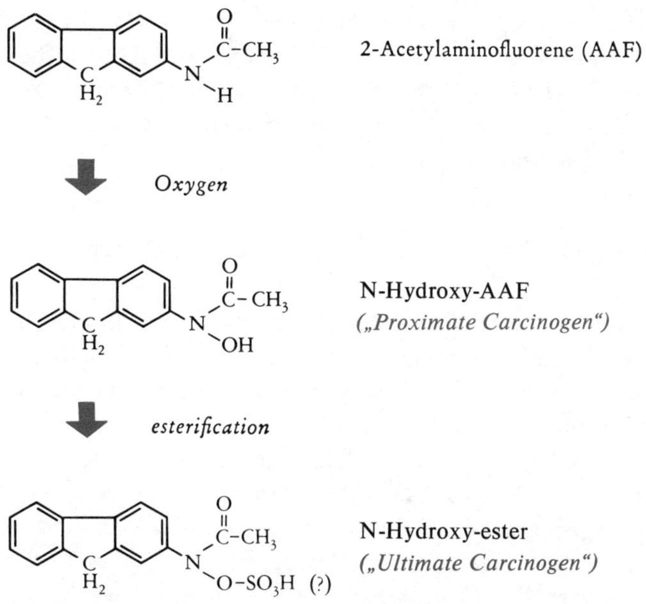

Activation to a carcinogen

Figure 6

products with AAF have been found in vivo. Thus, the connection between in vitro reactivity and in vivo carcinogenicity seems to have been established as firmly as is currently feasible.

The N-hydroxylation Hypothesis has its Difficulties

The pathway from simple amine to active ester is established in several cases, yet it is questionable whether it is obligatory. The Millers themselves do not consider the hydroxamic acid sulfate ester to be the final step for all the amines, although they do believe that this is the case for acetylaminofluorene. For amines such as the azo dyes and β-naphthylamine, the hydroxylamine seems to be sufficient as an "ultimate carcinogen." The case of the latter compound is particularly illuminating, since it is carcinogenic in the dog, even though the dog does not acetylate aromatic amines (Poirier).

N-hydroxylation in toto has been questioned to some extent by Arrhenius, who proposes that the radical intermediate leading to the

N-hydroxy derivative is to be seen as the ultimate carcinogen. This appears to be a moot point, however, for two reasons: experimental demonstration of its validity appears to be highly difficult, if not impossible; the N-hydroxy compounds *are present* as a result of amine metabolism and have been demonstrated to be more carcinogenic than their parent compounds.

Carcinogenic Aromatic Amines are Bound to Protein

The observation that MAB attacks methionine implies that the azo dyes are bound to protein, but the historical development was in fact the other way around. Already in 1947 the Millers had observed that the liver protein in rats who had been fed DAB turned pink in acid and yellow again in alkali. This color could not be extracted with organic solvents, but was obtained as amino acid-bound dye after digestion of the protein with proteolytic enzymes and hot alkali. Different dyes give different degrees of binding. 3'-Methyl-DAB is bound better than DAB, which in turn is bound much better than AB. Two questions seemed of prime importance after this discovery. What was the chemical nature of the binding? Does the binding have anything to do with the appearance of tumors?

Answers to the first question came only after the discovery of 3-CH₃S-MAB and the reactivity of N-benzoyloxy-MAB with amino acids other than methionine. Acting on this information, Lin and the Millers quickly showed that methionine and tyrosine are the amino acids primarily involved. Indications appeared that cysteine in protein also reacts.

The Stronger the Carcinogen, the Better the Binding to Protein

Whether the binding had anything to do with the appearance of tumors was a question which was tested quickly. DAB, AB, and 3'-methyl-DAB for example, are carcinogenic in the same order as that in which they bind to protein. Other C-monomethyl derivatives of DAB were also tested, and the rates at which DAB and its 5 C-monomethyl derivatives reached the maximum level of binding (about 4 weeks for DAB) were exactly correlated with their carcinogenic activities.

The hypothesis that binding to liver protein is a causative factor in liver carcinogenesis becomes quite well-founded, based not only on the above-mentioned results, but on the following:

a) If riboflavin is added to the diet of rats being fed DAB, both hepatoma production and protein-dye binding are suppressed.

b) Rats are sensitive to DAB, mice are not. Corresponding levels in binding of DAB to liver protein in the two species are also found.

c) The simultaneous feeding of 3-methylcholanthrene and DAB in the diet results again in suppression of both hepatomas and dye-protein binding.

All of these data thus made it appear that the production of liver tumors is dependent on whether azo dyes (DAB in particular) are bound to liver protein or not.

Carcinogenic Aromatic Amines are Bound Preferentially to h_2-Proteins

Numerous different proteins are present in the liver. The liver cell not only must maintain itself — it is also responsible for a whole series of "community projects." It must store glycogen in order to supply the entire organism with glucose in emergencies; nutrition transported in through the portal vein must be converted, broken down, and reassembled. Even a part of the body's heat production falls to the liver. Enzymes are necessary for all of these jobs, and all of these enzymes are proteins, thus explaining the plethora of liver proteins.

An effective method of separating the components of a protein mixture is electrophoresis. Proteins differ in their electrical charge, some being more negatively charged, others more positively. Proteins with no net charge are also found. If an electric field is applied to a protein solution, the positively charged proteins migrate to the negative pole, while the negatively charged proteins move toward the positive pole.

Such a separation can be accomplished on a column (zonal electrophoresis — see Figure 7). The proteins to be separated are placed on a column of, say, chemically modified cellulose, then subjected to an electric field. Usually the lower end of the column is made the positive pole, so that proteins migrate faster from the origin the more

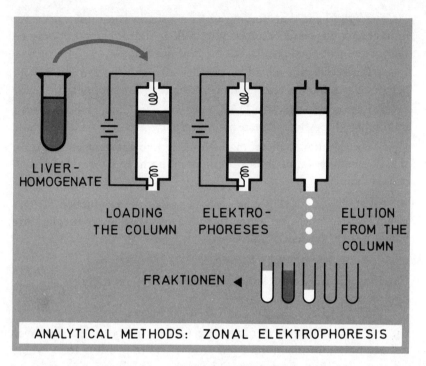

Figure 7

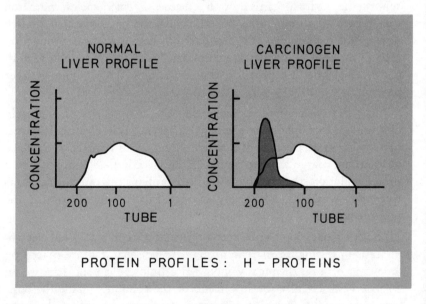

Figure 8

negatively charged they are. After an appropriate interval, the current is shut off, at which time the single protein fractions have at least been separated in zones. The column is eluted, and the zones are collected separately in test tubes (Figure 8).

Figure 8 shows a so-called elution diagram after electrophoresis of normal liver proteins. The transmission at 280 nm of each fraction (a measure of protein concentration) was measured, and this value was plotted on the ordinate. It is easy to see that these separations are not complete, but that there is a great deal of overlapping. Characteristic peaks have been assigned alphabetical classifications, with subpeaks receiving additional numbers.

Such an electrophoretogram was then carried out on the liver proteins from rats that had been fed the carcinogenic azo dye 3'-methyl-DAB (Sorof). Figure 8 shows the result of this experiment, in which not only the absorption at 280 nm (protein concentration), but also the absorption at 525 nm after addition of formic acid (dye concentration) was measured. The red area in the figure shows absorption at 525 nm, the white area at 280 nm. Dye thus appears predominantly in fractions 130—140, coincident with the so-called h_2-proteins.

h_2-Proteins are Greatly Reduced in Hepatomas

Protein analyses completely similar to those above were also carried out with liver tumors, in which it turned out that all of the hepatomas investigated (not simply azo dye induced hepatomas) contained much less h_2-protein than normal liver. The slowly growing Morris hepatomas, which closely resemble normal liver, are no exception.

This is an appropriate point to summarize the findings on the binding of carcinogenic azo dyes to liver proteins:

a) There is a clear correlation between carcinogenic activity and protein binding.

b) The dyes are preferably bound to a certain class of proteins — the so-called h_2-proteins.

c) These h_2-proteins, and the associated binding, are greatly reduced in hepatomas. A simple theory permits an easy interpretation of these data:

1. If h-proteins are growth-regulating proteins, then it is to be expected that these regulating substances are reduced in hepatomas.

2. All compounds that can react specifically with these proteins would then be carcinogens.

Soon after the Millers had originally discovered azo dye binding to liver protein and the lack of binding to hepatoma protein, they formulated this theory, now known as the "protein deletion hypothesis." Tumor cells differ from normal cells, according to this theory, in their lack of normal growth-regulating substances. Thus, the deletion of the h-proteins appears to be the decisive step in the cancerization of a liver cell. This conclusion has an immediate experimental consequence. If h-proteins are growth regulators, then it should be possible to inhibit the growth of certain cells with preparations of these proteins.

h_2-Proteins Inhibit the Growth of Cell Cultures (in vitro)

Sorof tried it, using HeLa cells (human tumor cells) and L-cells (derived from mouse fibroblasts). Enriched h-protein fractions were added to cultures of these cells, with the result that the growth of the cells really was inhibited. Moreover, this inhibition was reversible: when the h-proteins were washed out, the cells began to grow again. By this procedure, the trivial possibility was excluded that h-proteins were simply toxic and had killed off the cell cultures.

The h-protein story had reached its high point with this experiment. These proteins appeared to be at the center of the decisive conversion of a normal cell into a tumor cell. Then came the setbacks: after all, h-proteins really should only inhibit the growth of liver cells, for a liver growth regulator would have to be specific for liver. But neither HeLa nor L-cells are liver cells. People then suspected that Sorof's inhibition must have some kind of trivial explanation, and in fact it later turned out that the inhibitory effect of the h-proteins is associated with their arginase content. This enzyme cleaves arginine present in the nutrient medium, arginine which is necessary for cell growth, and so the cells starve. The addition of arginine compensated for the inhibitory effect of the h-proteins.

More bad news followed: the privileged place of the h-proteins was questioned in light of the observation that, in the nucleus, the carcinogenic dyes are bound primarily to albumin-like protein fractions. Finally, however — and this was really the hardest blow for believers in protein binding — it turned out that carcinogenic amines can also react with nucleic acids (Marroquin and Farber, Roberts and Warwick). With this observation we are confronted with the problem, which of these binding reactions is strategically important — to protein, RNA, or DNA. It remains true that the lion's share of the binding occurs to the h-proteins. There is apparently only one way to explain this high specificity in a trivial manner: h-proteins and activating enzymes must be identical; the activated, reactive azo dye derivatives would react with their nearest neighbors, that is, with these enzymes. So far, however, there has been no success in confirming even this hypothesis (Sorof, Ketterer). We can say simply that, at the moment, no one has any idea of what the function of the h_2-protein might be.

Binding of carcinogens to DNA plays hardly any role, quantitatively, but it "fits" beautifully into the theoretical models of modern biology. Thus, the remarkable ability of tumor cells to "give birth to tumor cells continually" even when no external carcinogen is present is easily explained: any change in the genetic material — the DNA — must necessarily be transmitted to the daughter cells. Tumor cells must, therefore, differ genetically from the corresponding normal cells, an apparently necessary conclusion. In fact, it is only convenient. Further remarks on this point and on recent research on DNA and cancer will be found in a separate chapter on this subject (page 193).

Summary

Carcinogenic aromatic amines (N,N-dimethyl-4-aminoazobenzene and other aminoazo dyes, β-naphthylamine, benzidine, 2-acetylaminofluorene) are activated to their effective forms via hydroxylation. Such oxidation can take place on the aromatic ring or on the amino group. The N-hydroxylation appears to play the most important role: N-hydroxyamines (amides) are in most cases better and more versatile carcinogens than their parent amines; they have been designated "proximate carcinogens" by the Millers. Esterification products of N-hydroxy amides react in the test tube with cell components, such as methionine. In the cell itself, sulfate esters might be the actual active forms of carcinogenic aromatic amides. For those cases in which amines appear to be more carcinogenic than the corresponding amides, or in animals in which the amides are not formed, the N-hydroxy amine appears to be the "ultimate carcinogen."

Carcinogenic aromatic amines are preferentially bound to a particular class of soluble proteins (h-proteins). Carcinogenicity and protein binding are well correlated, and the h-proteins are severely reduced in hepatomas. The "deletion hypothesis" requires that the h-proteins have a growth-regulating effect. The loss of these proteins would then directly cause uncontrolled growth into tumors. Treatment of cell cultures with h-protein preparations did lead to reversible growth inhibition. However, contaminating arginase was found to be the active principle, by removing the arginine necessary for cell growth.

Carcinogenic aromatic amines react not only with protein, but also with nucleic acids. The binding to DNA is now believed to be a decisive step for carcinogenesis.

A CLOSER LOOK AT CHEMICAL
CARCINOGENESIS: QUANTITATIVE ASPECTS

"I contend, however, that in each particular natural theory there is only so much real science as there is mathematics," said Kant years before Lord Kelvin. And with this severe criterion he dismissed the chemistry of his time: "... thus chemistry can never become more than systematic art or an experimental doctrine; it can never become true science." Chemistry has long since matured beyond Kant's verdict, with the firm theoretical underpinnings of thermodynamics and atomic theory.

Even the biology of our time and scientific medicine are more and more to be considered as exact science. The fascination with the phenomenon of living things is still an important driving force of biological research, but *vis vitalis* and *vis regenerativa* have been bid farewell, with regrets and relief simultaneously. Simple DNA molecules have won the race, and the rational language of cybernetics today dominates such basic biological phenomena as inheritance and adaptation. Cancer research, to be sure, remained in large degree a "systematic art," and we have not yet been as successful in building a generally valid and generally accepted structure of ideas. Still, cancerology has not completely given up on mathematics: quantitative investigations into chemical carcinogenesis gave the primary impetus to a "mathematical theory" of tumor development.

For a long time people had been satisfied with classifying a substance as a good or poor carcinogen. Even in 1948, Badger was still using a simple semiquantitative system for the classification of chemical carcinogens:

very strong	carcinogen	+ + + +
strong	carcinogen	+ + +
moderate	carcinogen	+ +
weak	carcinogen	+
inactive	carcinogen	0

Here, too, Badger had to admit that, because of the difficulties of biological testing, the accuracy could very well vary by one "cross" in evaluation. This would mean, then, that on repeat of a carcinogenicity test, a compound could be classified as either a weak carcinogen or as inactive altogether. The decision as to whether a substance is really noncarcinogenic is extremely difficult, and again and again new investigations with more animals and higher doses are forcing revisions. The recent hot discussion about the Pill and artificial sweeteners (estrogen and cyclamates) illustrates how careful one must be with "final decisions." The problem of borderline activity is fundamentally insoluble.

What is soluble, at least in principle, is the problem of substituting quantitative indicators of activity for the previous qualitative indices. Many authors have invented their own systems (Berenblum and the Millers, for example), but the most well-known example is the so-called Iball Index, proposed by the American Iball in 1939.

The Iball Index

Let us consider two examples in skin carcinogenesis: mice of the same age, sex, and strain are divided into groups of about 30 mice. A 0.3 percent solution of the compound to be tested is dropped onto the shaved backs of the mice; the solvent might be benzene (previously common), although acetone is now known to have less effect on the skin. This painting is repeated twice a week until the first papillomas (warts) are visible and can be counted. The following table outlines such an experiment with two different organic compounds: (Table 2).

Table 2: Parameters of Carcinogenic Activity

Compound	% Tumor-bearing Mice	Average Latent Period	Iball Index
DMBA	65	43	157
1,2,5,6-Dibenzacridine	24	350	7

The two substances obviously have very different behavior: DMBA induces tumors on the average after only 43 days, affecting 65 percent of the mice. Dibenzacridine induces tumors in only 24 percent of the mice, requiring almost a year latent period.

A "good" carcinogen is characterizable in two ways:

1. It can induce tumors in more animals than a "poor" carcinogen.

2. It induces tumors within a shorter time.

This means that tumor yield, as well as latent period, can be a measure of carcinogenic activity. Then Iball proposed the following quotient as a carcinogenesis index:

$$I_{Carc} = \frac{\text{Tumor yield } (\%)}{\text{Latent period (days)}} \times 100 = \frac{A}{L} \times 100,$$

where the factor 100 simply serves to turn out whole numbers. Quantities calculated in this fashion are shown in the last column of Table 2.

Obviously, these numbers are valid only in the applied system: the indices of this example are applicable only for mice of a given strain, and the compounds must be "painted" on the skin. If by chance one wanted to compare the abilities of these two compounds to induce sarcomas in rats after subcutaneous injection, he could then probably count on different carcinogenic activities and different indices. DMBA, for example, is an excellent skin carcinogen in mice, but only an average sarcoma inducer in rats. Similarly, it should be self-evident that it is insufficient to simply compare 0.3 percent solutions of carcinogens: a strong carcinogen is effective at low doses, whereas a weak carcinogen must be given at high concentrations. Thus, there is the danger of underestimating strong carcinogens, if one limits himself to a single concentration. For this reason, the necessity of establishing a dose-response relationship for each carcinogen is unavoidable.

All in all, Boyland placed the use of the Iball Index in perspective by noting that it offers about as much information as a single number could offer concerning the desirable attributes of a Playboy Playmate.

Dose-Response Curves

Many months can pass between the injection of a carcinogen and eventual development of a palpable tumor. In spite of this, exact dose-response curves can be determined even for carcinogenic activities provided that biological variables (species, strain, sex, age, diet, etc.) are held constant.

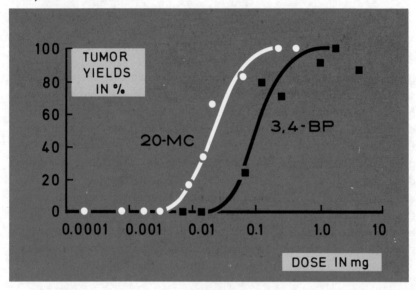

Figure 9

Figure 9 reproduces an example studied by Bryan and Shimkin: increasing quantities of the carcinogenic hydrocarbons indicated were injected subcutaneously in mice, and the sarcomas arising at the site of the single injection were counted. It is seen that 0.1 mg of methyl-cholanthrene suffices to produce a 100 percent sarcoma yield, but that about ten times as much benzpyrene is required for the same effect.

Usually tumors cannot be induced by a one-time treatment of the animals. As a rule, feeding over a long time period is necessary to induce, for example, liver cancer. Yet even in cases of "chronic" feeding, one finds quite strict mathematical relationships. Take for example the case of induction of hepatomas in rats using DAB (see p. 24), an example quantitatively analyzed in 1948 by Druckrey and Kuepfmueller. The following table summarizes their results:

Table 3: Induction of Liver Cancer by Daily Feeding of N,N-dimethyl-4-aminoazobenzene (DAB)

Daily Dose of DAB	Latent Period (Days)	Total Dose
30	34	1020
20	52	1040
10	95	950
5	190	950
3	350	1050
1	700	700

The last column of this table is surprising: whether the daily dose was 3 mg or 30 mg/rat, the total dose of DAB required to induce hepatomas amounted in each case to about 1 gram. At lower daily doses about a year was required to reach the total dose; at high doses liver tumors were obtained after one month. This finding can be expressed in the formula $D = d \times t$, in which D = total dose, d = daily dose, and t = time.

The effect of DAB (tumor induction), therefore, is dependent on the summation of all the single doses ("summation effect"). "These results make it plain that the primary carcinogenic effects of all single doses, no matter how small, are retained and add up *irreversibly* over the life span of the rat to 'tumor induction' (Druckrey)."

Carcinogenic Effects are Irreversible

Apparently a tissue — or more correctly, the cells of a tissue — cannot recover from the "carcinogenic effects" of a chemical carcinogen. If "recovery processes" were to play a decisive role, then it should not be inconsequential how long a carcinogen is fed in any given case: for long feeding periods (low doses), recovery reactions ought be more clearly apparent than for short feeding periods. Since in spite of varying latent periods the same total dosage is reached, such reactions are out of the question; the effect of DAB on liver cells is therefore "irreversible."

DAB is hardly an isolated case. Numerous investigations have confirmed again and again that carcinogenic effects are irreversible. Simply the fact that tumors can be induced with a single application (as with subcutaneous injection of carcinogenic hydrocarbons) points in this direction, but even in chronic testing this irreversibility can be convincingly demonstrated. In one such experiment Schmähl tested a more recent carcinogen, dimethylaminostilbene, which induces ear duct tumors in rats with uncanny precision. These growths become palpable in all of the animals of an experimental group "simultaneously" (within a 5-day range).

A collection of rats was given a daily dose of 1 mg/kg regularly until the occurrence of ear duct tumors. Another collection received weekly in alternation double the dose, 2 mg/kg per day, or normal feed, so that the total doses in the two series were the same. If recovery processes from the cancerogenic process are possible, then these could proceed in the weeks without treatment, and the total dose necessary for tumor induction ought to be greater in the group with the alternated feedings than for continuous administration of the compound. This was, however, not the case: the mean total doses in the two groups were practically equal, and amounted in the continuous experiment to 373 ± 75 mg/kg and in the alternating experiment 348 ± 70 mg/kg, so that in this experimental system, too, the irreversibility of the cancerogenic effect could be demonstrated (Schmähl).

Thus, summation effects and irreversibility characterize chemical carcinogenesis, which, however, is still not sufficiently quantitatively described by these concepts. Time itself is important and appears to play a role independent of the carcinogen in tumor induction.

Carcinogenesis as an Accelerated Process

Even in the quantitative analysis of tumor induction from DAB (Table 3), it is striking that at very small doses (1 mg/kg) the total dose required for tumor induction is significantly reduced. Instead of 950 to 1050 mg, only 700 mg are required. This reduction in the total dose accompanying smaller daily doses appears much more clearly in the use of certain carcinogens other than DAB. For diethylnitrosamine — another liver carcinogen — the total dose falls over the entire range of daily doses; the smaller the daily dose, the smaller the total dose. Thus, the formula given for DAB ($D = d \cdot t$) is no longer valid. Instead, the following approximation is much more nearly correct: $d \times t^2 = $ constant. That is, the daily doses are not simply summed over time to a constant total dose. This means that time itself plays a role in carcinogenesis, that time supplies its own contribution to tumor formation.

In this connection the terms "amplification" and "accelerated reactions" have been used, and in fact the latter equation resembles a well-known formula from classical physics describing free fall:

$$S = \frac{g}{2} \times t^2$$

where $S = $ distance of fall, $g = $ acceleration due to gravity, and $t = $ time of fall. These concepts from mechanics are easily transferred to the context of carcinogenesis: t would correspond to the time of feeding, $g/2$ to the daily dose, and, finally, S would be equated to the "distance to the tumor," a distance that is naturally covered more quickly according to the "accelerating force."

According to this picture, a carcinogen is a "force," which is constantly affecting the target cell. In mechanics a constant force leads to accelerated motion, and chemical carcinogenesis thus by simple analogy appears to be an "accelerated process."

Physical laws also require that, even after removal of the effective force, motion does not stop; only the acceleration is lost, and the

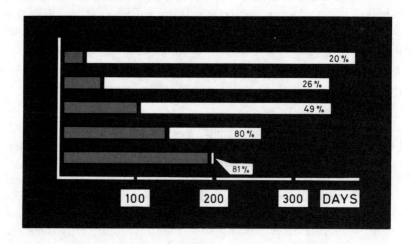

Figure 10

body continues to move with a constant velocity. By transference of these relationships to carcinogenesis, it would follow that tumors develop even when feeding of the carcinogen is only for a limited time. Figure 10 shows such a "Stop-Experiment," carried out by Druckrey again with DAB. This experiment shows again that the carcinogenic effect is irreversible, for even after removal of the carcinogen, the effect of the compound is not nullified. To be sure, fewer hepatomas appear later and later, the shorter the feeding period, but this is to be expected; if the accelerating long-term feeding is stopped, the carcinogenesis must go on at a constant rate.

It must logically be entirely possible to set the carcinogenic process in motion with a single "shove" (a physicist would speak of momentum), and this is also the case. We have already pointed out several cases in which tumors have been induced after a single treatment with a carcinogen.

Thus, it is entirely justifiable to conceive of carcinogenesis as an accelerated process related to the accelerated motion of classical mechanics. Yet tumor induction and free fall are two basically different systems, and we will soon come up against the limits of this analogy.

There are no Subthreshold Carcinogenic Doses

Let us return once more to the induction of hepatomas with diethylnitrosamine. We have already mentioned the existence of the following connection between daily dose and latent period: $dt^n =$ constant. If we take the logarithm of this expression, we obtain $\log d = \text{constant} - n \log t$. This equation simply says that one must obtain a straight line if d (daily dose) and t (latent period) are plotted on a log-log graph. Figure 11 shows that this equation is strictly followed. The experimental points lie on a line, even down to very small daily doses, permitting an important conclusion: there is no reason to assume that sufficiently small doses fail to induce cancer. To put it another way: there is no subthreshold carcinogenic dose. Granted, at very low doses the latent periods would be longer than the natural lifetimes of the animals, and the rats would die a natural death without having developed tumors.

From the slope of the line on the log-log plot, the exponent n of the above equations can be determined. In this case, $n = 2.3$, so that

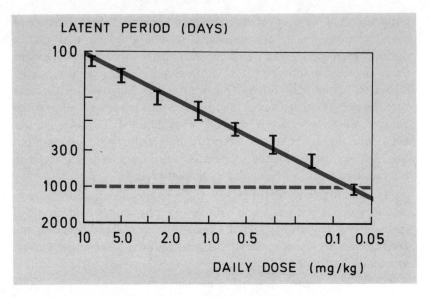

Figure 11

for diethylnitrosamine-induced hepatocellular carcinomas, $dt^{2.3} =$ constant. The agreement with the "acceleration theory" is rather good, and other nitrosamines also fit. For di-n-propyl-nitrosamine $n = 2.2$, and for N-nitroso-sarcosine esters, 2.5 was obtained. For certain other carcinogens, however, n is much greater than 2.

Carcinogens Differ in their Acceleration Behavior

Let us now put a few carcinogens side by side and compare their exponents n for the above equation. DAB, as we established at the beginning of this discussion, follows a pure summation law, not counting the very lowest dosages. The same total dose of carcinogen must be obtained independently of the latent period. This independence of time means that $n = 1$.

For dimethylaminostilbene, n is calculated to be 3.0; benzpyrene has a "slope" of 4.0 when painted three times weekly. Some carcinogenic hydrocarbons have given values as high as 4.7 on subcutaneous injection.

Experience with human tumors also fits: Nordling established that cancer mortality increases with the 6th power of age, using general cancer statistics from England, France, Norway, and the United States. Doll reported similar findings obtained from analysis of lung cancer cases in smokers; here, too, mortality increases with the 5th or 6th power of time. "This proves," Druckrey writes, "that carcinogenesis due to prolonged exposure follows the same dose-response and the same time relationships, whether in animal experiments or in human statistics" (Table 4).

Table 4: The Role of Time in Chemical Carcinogenesis

Compound	Acceleration Factors Species	Organ	n
DAB	rat	liver	1.1
Di-n-butylnitrosamine	rat	bladder	1.4
Diethylnitrosamine	rat	liver	2.3
N-Nitrososarcosine-ethyl ester	rat	esophagus	2.5
Dimethylaminostilbene	rat	ear duct	3.0
3,4-Benzpyrene	mouse	skin	4.0

Biological Significance of Acceleration

Newtonian acceleration, such as assumed above, is incompatible with the higher exponents of the dose-latency period equation. This is not too surprising, since the system cell-organism-carcinogen bears only a superficial resemblance to Galileo's freely falling bodies. Let us imagine a few possibilities for explaining acceleration in carcinogenesis:

1. Let us assume that a carcinogen basically has two effects: the induction of tumor cells and their multiplication. Assuming certain limiting conditions, this leads naturally to a law of the type $D = dt^n$.

2. At low doses and correspondingly long latent periods, the time for tumor development reaches into the animals' old age, which means a greater risk of cancer. We will discuss later what this increased risk can mean biologically. In the present connection it could explain why cumulatively less carcinogen is required with longer latent periods.

3. One could imagine that "time" has a similar "effect" to that of a carcinogen. For example, carcinogens induce cell division, but such division takes place anyway in the tissue. Thus, the longer the latent period, the more "natural" cell divisions, and the less carcinogen required.

4. Essentially all carcinogens are toxic, i. e., they can kill cells. This means that especially at high daily doses cells are lost from the

system. In other words, the carcinogen is getting in its own way. With high daily doses then, more carcinogen would be needed than with low doses.

5. If the toxic effect of a carcinogen is primarily against normal cells, that means that "resistant" tumor cells are favored in selection by the carcinogen. This selection could also contribute to acceleration.

Just these few examples demonstrate how complicated interactions can be in the system cell-organism-carcinogen, and how complicated the temporal dependence of tumor induction must be. Let us give up on a mathematical treatment of this problem and finish the chapter by returning to the question of what makes a "good" carcinogen.

Latent Periods and Tumor Yields are not Necessarily Coupled

As we have now shown several times, a good carcinogen can induce many tumors in a short time at low doses. Consequently, it was tacitly assumed that high tumor yields and short latent periods mean the same thing. Yet as more and more experience was gained in chemical carcinogenesis, it more and more turned out that latent periods and tumor yields by no means need to be coupled. This means, however, that the carcinogenic effect of, say, an unsaturated polycyclic hydrocarbon consists of at least two components, of which one determines the number of resulting tumors, and the other establishes the time required until these tumors become manifest. These two carcinogenic components are especially easily separated in the induction of skin tumors in the mouse; thus, we must now turn to this special area of skin carcinogenesis.

Summary

In spite of long latent periods for tumor development, there are exact dose-response relationships. From these relationships we find no reason to believe that there is a threshold for chemical carcinogens, below which they have no more effect.

The effects of chemical carcinogens are irreversible. Even time makes a "unique contribution" to carcinogenesis, in that acceleration is usually found instead of simple addition of daily doses.

Latent periods and tumor yields need not be coupled.

MULTIPLE STEP HYPOTHESIS OF CHEMICAL CARCINOGENESIS

Since Yamagiwa's pioneer experiments on the rabbit's ear, the skin has again and again been the organ of choice for experiments in "artificial" carcinogenesis. The reasons are obvious: skin is easily accessible, and a pipette is sufficient to apply any given carcinogenic substance. Just as important is the fact that one can look at the tumors. Palpation or autopsy are unnecessary; careful visual observation is enough to establish whether and how many tumors have developed on the back of a mouse or on the ear of a rabbit.

The Berenblum-Mottram Experiment: Two Steps Lead to Papillomas

In order to induce skin tumors, it is usual to paint 0.1 ml of a 0.3 percent acetone solution of methylcholanthrene, benzpyrene, or dimethylbenzanthracene (DMBA) on the shaved backs of mice one or more times a week. One can also succeed in inducing papillomas and carcinomas with a single large dose, although the yield is then only moderate. In addition to these "classical" methods, one can also arrive at skin tumors by a more refined route:

1. The mice are first painted or fed a dose of carcinogenic hydrocarbon (25 µg on the back or 1 mg by feeding) insufficient to induce tumors during the normal life span of the mice.

2. These mice are then treated weekly on the back with a 0.5 percent solution of croton oil (a seed oil from the tropical plant *Croton tiglium*), until the first papillomas become visible after about 8 weeks. If only croton oil is applied, without a previous treatment with a carcinogen, no papillomas appear. Thus, croton oil is not a carcinogen under these conditions.

This experiment was first reported by Mottram and later refined and extensively applied by Berenblum. It shows that the combination of two noncarcinogenic events can lead to tumors:

1. Subthreshold single dose   2. Noncarcinogenic
    of a carcinogen   +   croton oil   → Tumor.

A comparison with the photographic process is apparent: light *can* cause an image on a light-sensitive plate after extensive exposure. Normally, however, the plate is only exposed for a short period ("subthreshold dose"), in order to induce a latent image, and the exposure is followed by chemical development of the activated silver salt grains to visible grains of metallic silver. Thus, in principle, the combination of subthreshold illumination plus chemical development leads to the same end result as an extended exposure alone.

The so-called Berenblum-Mottram experiment can thus be interpreted in the following manner: DMBA or some other carcinogenic hydrocarbon induces *latent* tumor cells, which then develop to tumors under the influence of croton oil. The induction of the latent tumor cells is usually called *initiation;* the induction of an actual gross tumor is *promotion.* Initiation would thus be analogous to the subthreshold-illumination of a photographic plate, while chemical development would correspond to the effect of croton oil (promotion).

If we were to develop a photographic plate first, and then expose it, we would obviously get no picture. Berenblum undertook an analogous experiment with croton oil and carcinogenic hydrocarbon, and found that, in the reverse two-step induction procedure, no tumors are induced.

Not Only Croton Oil can Promote

Although croton oil led to the discovery of promotion of latent tumor cells, it is by no means the only substance that will do this. Others are Tween (a detergent), anthralin (1,8,9-trihydroxyanthracene), and various phenols. "Complete carcinogens" can apparently both initiate and promote (carcinogenic hydrocarbons, for example), but if given only once in low dosage, their effect is restricted to initiation.

The two-step hypothesis permits a prediction: there must be substances which can only initiate and not promote — these would be the actual complements to croton oil. Such a substance has been discovered: for mouse skin, urethane (ethyl carbamate) is a pure initiator. Mice that are treated with urethane and painted on the back for several weeks with croton oil develop papillomas. Urethane alone, even with continuous administration, does not cause skin tumors. Thus, it is possible to induce tumors with a combination of two apparently noncarcinogenic substances.

Irritation and Carcinogenesis

How did Berenblum actually arrive at the two-step hypothesis? He did not start with quantitative considerations about latent periods or tumor yields, but simply approached the question of whether irritation per se has anything to do with carcinogenesis.

Most carcinogens are substances which irritate tissue in high enough doses so that this is a pertinent question. People were actually convinced that there is a clear relationship between tissue irritation and tumor induction. Irritation in the skin is manifested in hyperplasia (see Figure 52): increased cell division acts to replace the damaged cells. Thus, the question becomes: does carcinogenesis have anything to do with hyperplasia? Let us listen to Berenblum himself:

> At first, various simple irritants were tested on the skin of mice for evidence of carcinogenic action. They all induced hyperplasia but not tumours. It seemed clear, then, that irritation per se could not be held responsible for carcinogenic action.
>
> Then, various noncarcinogenic irritants were applied together with a carcinogen in order to determine whether extra irritation intensified carcinogenic action. The results were confusing: some irritants, notably mustard gas (the poison gas of World War I), and cantharidin, when applied in very dilute solutions (sufficient only to induce very mild skin irritation) caused a dramatic inhibition of carcinogenic action (i. e., eliciting an anticarcinogenic effect); other irritants, notably the drug croton oil, caused a striking augmentation of carcinogenic action (i. e., eliciting a cocarcinogenic effect); while most other irritants had no influence one way or the other. It seemed, therefore, that irritating action was not a critical factor for carcinogenesis even as an adjuvant.

Berenblum, however, proceeded one step further:

> The next phase of the inquiry was to replace the carcinogen by a noncarcinogenic irritant during part of the course of treatment only ... Croton oil was chosen as the irritant, and it was found that when the substance was applied for several months before the carcinogenic treatment, there was no speeding up of tumour development or any increase in tumour yield, whereas when it was applied after a somewhat inadequate course of carcinogenic treatment, there was a striking increase in tumour yield.

This experiment was the immediate predecessor (in protocol) of Mottram's experiment, which as the last logical step in the progression of experimental systems directly led to the proposition that skin carcinogenesis is a two-step process. Lung tumors may also be induced by a procedure which, operationally at least, consists of two steps. Before we look at this experimental procedure closer, however, we still have to come back to Berenblum's original question: does carcinogenesis have anything to do with irritation, or, in the special case of skin carcinogenesis, does tumor evocation have anything to do with hyperplasia?

The question must be made more precise; we must distinguish whether hyperplasia has anything to do with initiation or promotion. The urethane experiments have at least given one clear answer: hyperplasia is *not* necessary for the formation of latent tumor cells. After urethane feeding, no damage to the epidermis was noted, and correspondingly no repair processes.

The findings for promotion are much less clear. In this connection, the work of Hecker and his coworkers has become important: they have succeeded in isolating and elucidating the structure of several active principles from croton oil. Using one of these compounds (called TPA by Hecker), it was possible to carry out two-step carcinogenesis experiments on an exact quantitative basis. TPA is not only a promoter, it is strongly inflammatory (2 µg applied to the mouse's back induces one big "burn blister" under the skin — an "edema," in medical language), as well as hyperplastic.

The phorbol esters offer rational possibilities for solving this problem: the exact knowledge of their molecular structures permits one to make precisely defined changes in this molecule and thus to probe which components of the structure help to determine its biological activity. In such experiments one might succeed in finding compounds which are only inflammatory or only promoting. After all, "pure" agents with "purely" cocarcinogenic effects were also unknown until now.

Rous Discovers the Two-Step Process in the Rabbit's Ear

At the time (1941) that Berenblum published his first experiments with croton oil on mouse skin, Rous reported observations on rabbit ears which led him to the same conclusions. The decisive experiments were the following:

1. If the ears of rabbits were treated with tar, tumors developed. If the tar treatment was interrupted, the tumors disappeared in many

cases. When tar treatment was begun again, the tumors could appear in the exact same positions.

2. Renewed tar painting was not the only thing that would reawaken the lost tumors: treatment with turpentine or chloroform, which are non-carcinogenic, could also cause a spurt in the stopped tumor growth. Simple wound healing also sufficed. By punching a hole in the ear with a cork borer, Rous caused tumors to grow at the wound.

Again the conclusion was reached that (at least) two processes lead to tumor development:

a) The induction of latent tumor cells

b) The propagation of these latent cells into tumors by noncarcinogenic events.

Croton Oil is not a "Chemical Cork Borer"

Rous's observation that simple wound healing after mechanical injury decisively accelerates tumor growth could be taken to mean that croton oil is to be conceived as a "chemical cork borer." According to this idea, croton oil simply caused a wound, the healing of which represented the actual cocarcinogenic effect. This conception is contradicted, however, by the knowledge that many inflammatory substances which lead to regenerative hyperplasia ("wound healing") are not cocarcinogenic.

Morphologic investigation of skin treated with TPA also indicates a specific effect: the first effect is not a wound, a loss of epidermal cells. First the basal cells swell, including the nuclei, followed by notable cell multiplication (hyperplasia). The multiple cell divisions do not take place to close a wound, but rather, in a sense, from a "standstill." Only later is there a sloughing off of entire cell layers, i. e., real wounding.

Two Steps are an Insufficient Description

Boutwell has succeeded in further dividing the promotion phase — the development of latent tumor cells. Mice were initiated with DMBA, then treated with croton oil and turpentine. The following diagram indicates the details (Figure 12).

Thus, turpentine can replace certain "late effects" of croton oil, but not early effects. That is, turpentine can obviously continue

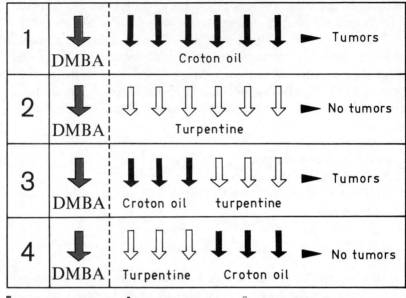

1 DMBA Croton oil ► Tumors

2 DMBA Turpentine ► No tumors

3 DMBA Croton oil turpentine ► Tumors

4 DMBA Turpentine Croton oil ► No tumors

⬇=DMBA-Initiation ↓ = Croton oil ⇩ = Turpentine
application application

Figure 12

promotion to the finish, but cannot start it. Boutwell has proposed the name "conversion" for the first portion of promotion, indicating that potential tumor cells are changed at this stage into actual latent tumor cells, which are then propagated to gross tumors. It is probable that non specific hyperplasia or wound healing can act as a propagator, but not a converter.

Promotion is Reversible

The interval between successive croton oil treatments is by no means unimportant. If a given total dose of croton oil (1.5 mg) is divided into exceedingly small doses given frequently, or into doses of a standard effective level given at increasingly larger intervals, either change results in a large reduction in tumor yield (Boutwell).

This means that the effect of croton oil is reversible, in contrast to the results of similar experiments carried out with DMBA, in which the additivity mentioned earlier is the rule.

Initiation is Irreversible

The time one waits before beginning croton oil treatment after initiation has little effect. Latent period and tumor yield remain the same, whether promotion is begun immediately or 40 weeks later. This means that the initiated cells are retained and, so to speak, are waiting for a signal from croton oil. This stability is really astounding, for in the course of 40 weeks the population of epidermal cells is often replaced, and the cell generation which was treated with carcinogen has long since given way to younger cells. The changed information content of the potential tumor cells must have been passed on many times.

This is hardly a compelling conclusion, for it could easily be the case that the changed cells simply lie there, excluded from the constant cell regeneration. Although this alternative appears somewhat ad hoc, it becomes more probable after one is aware of the exact mechanism of resupply of epidermal cells. Figure 13 indicates two model systems which differ in the spatial orientation of the mitoses. Model (B) would easily explain why the same number of tumor foci remain after a long time and, correspondingly, why the same tumor yields are attained even after a year. This model has one slight disadvantage: it is probably entirely incorrect.

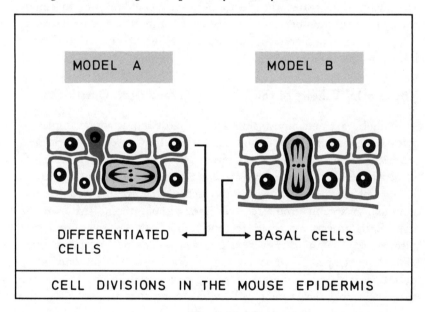

Figure 13

Model (A) is more probable, for "squeezed-out" cells (as shown in the sketch) have actually been observed under the microscope (Iversen). Bullough also reported that he could show that, in the mouse epidermis, the plane of a mitosis as a rule is so oriented that both daughter cells remain in the basal cell layer: "It may be only the increasing pressure that ultimately squeezes cells into the more distal layers where keratin synthesis begins." Autoradiographic studies also support model (A). Iversen, for example, labeled epidermal cells with tritiated thymidine (thus marking those cells in the S-phase) and followed the migration of the label. It turned out that only 10 percent of the labeled cells immediately migrated to the upper cell layers and that the predominant portion of the labeled basal cells simply remains in the basal cell layer after mitosis. Karatschai confirmed this finding with the new method of relief autoradiography.

Model (A) could also explain why the number of latent tumor cells does not change (on the average) with time. One would expect, however, that occasional latent tumor cells become completely lost by pressure to the surface or that more than the average number of latent tumor cells remain, simply because by chance they do not get pushed out. In short, the longer one waits before beginning croton oil treatment, the greater the fluctuations one could expect in tumor yield, i. e., the number of tumor-bearing animals ought to decrease. This has been observed in one instance, out of four experiments known to the authors.

The General Validity of the Two-Step Hypothesis is Questionable

Rabbit ears and mouse skin are the most important examples of two-step experiments, but they are not the only cases. Huggins once made the following remarkable observation: rats of a strain in which spontaneous sarcomas are never found were given subcutaneous injections of sesame oil (a frequently used vehicle for fat-soluble compounds). A second group received methylcholanthrene (MC) in the diet. Both groups remained free of tumors. If, however, rats that received MC in the diet were also given sesame oil injections, these animals developed sarcomas at the injection site. The obvious interpretation is that the dietary carcinogen converted some connective tissue cells to latent tumor cells, which were then promoted by the irritation due to the injection.

Nonetheless, tumor induction according to the two-step scheme does not appear to be generally applicable experimentally. The development of leukemias seems to fit, but in contrast there is yet no good system for inducing hepatomas in a two-step fashion. Even mouse skin is not simply mouse skin: the tail is refractory to continuous treatment with DMBA, while in the mouse's *ear*, the combination of feeding DMBA and painting TPA fails to lead to tumors. In rats, the standard two-step procedure on the back simply does not work.

If DMBA or (recently) diethylnitrosamine in subthreshold doses is injected into hamsters, followed by respiration of iron oxide dust (hematite), bronchial carcinomas develop. "Noncarcinogenic" sulfur dioxide was equally successful as an active agent in the second step.

Syncarcinogenesis: Carcinogens can Substitute for Each Other

The discovery of the many varied chemical carcinogens had quickly led to the question of whether all of these substances set in motion a common mechanism leading to development of tumors. Carcinogens appear in many different chemical classes, such as the polycyclic aromatic hydrocarbons, the aromatic amines, and the nitrosamines. Urethane is a minimal combination of both amide and ester, and thiourea is urea with a sulfur in place of the usual oxygen.

This multiplicity of physicochemical properties hinted that, as an example, the induction of hepatomas with DAB or diethylnitrosamine (DENA) takes place in two entirely different manners. Yet this suspicion was directly contradicted by experiment. When both carcinogens were fed simultaneously, only 60 percent of the doses required separately were necessary to induce tumors (Schmähl). Thus, DENA can substitute for DAB to a considerable extent.

This finding is hardly an isolated case. In the 1930's and 1940's, Hieger and Rush had already found that 3,4-benzpyrene and DMBA are exchangeable. Friedrich-Freksa (1940) described how methylcholanthrene can substitute for benzpyrene and vice versa. To be sure, it seems entirely plausible that closely related substances such as the hydrocarbons should be exchangeable in this fashion. Yet even the very different compounds 4-nitroquinoline-*N*-oxide and 3-methylcholanthrene can substitute for each other in skin carcinogenesis (Nakahara).

Especially surprising were successful attempts to induce skin cancer by simultaneous treatment with chemical carcinogen and radiation. Hoshino et al. administered subthreshold doses of 4-nitroquinoline-*N*-oxide and ^{90}Sr β-radiation simultaneously and obtained papillomas, fibrosarcomas, and carcinomas. Hence, the authors concluded that the effects induced by 4-nitroquinoline-N-oxide and β-radiation are qualitatively equivalent.

Schmähl too had concluded from his experiments: "The addition of the carcinogenic effects compels the assumption that the site of attack of the carcinogenic effect must take place in the same place in the cell; if this were not so, then the addition is not understandable." (In Hoshino's case, there is one significant detail. It is *not* irrelevant whether 4-nitroquinoline-N-oxide is administered before or after the radiation.)

It is entirely possible that the replaceability of the carcinogenic stimuli does not hold true for the entire course of carcinogenesis. In the Berenblum and Rous terminology this could mean that different carcinogens have completely different primary effects, but that they share a common property in their ability to promote.

Syncarcinogenesis and Cocarcinogenesis: More than a Question of Semantics

The two concepts of syncarcinogenesis (K. H. Bauer) and cocarcinogenesis are only superficially synonymous. Syncarcinogenesis refers to synergistic action of carcinogens, while cocarcinogenesis refers to measures that assist carcinogenesis but which in themselves need not be carcinogenic. Croton oil is an example of a cocarcinogenic substance which in itself is not carcinogenic.

In the strict sense, croton oil is not noncarcinogenic; at high dosages one obtains a significant number of papillomas. Croton oil is a mixture of many substances, and there was the possibility that the promoting and carcinogenic properties could be assigned to different materials. For just this reason Hecker undertook the fractionation of croton oil in order to isolate and characterize pure compounds. Even this did not answer the original question, for the pure "promoters" still revealed a weak carcinogenic property at high dosage.

As a result, it has occasionally been concluded that the two-step experiment is really only a special case of syncarcinogenesis, that we see "only" an interaction of different carcinogens, differing only in that a potentiating, instead of additive, effect is seen. According to this view, there is no fundamental difference between initiation and promotion.

This, however, is a crass denial of the facts already discussed above, that initiation is irreversible and that promotion is not. In addition, the sequence of application — as stated above — determines whether tumors arise. Croton oil treatment *before* application of carcinogen is without effect. Finally, the ostensibly carcinogenic effects of croton oil and its pure components can be conveniently discussed under the table: it is experimentally impossible to exclude spontaneous initiation due to, say, UV irradiation or cosmic rays. Croton oil simply promotes these spontaneously induced latent tumor cells.

Summary

The chemical induction of papillomas can be dissected into two phases in the mouse skin system. The first phase (initiation) induces so-called latent tumor cells; the second (promotion) propagates these cells into tumors.

Promotion is possible with noncarcinogenic substances, of which croton oil is the best known example. Initiation is irreversible, promotion reversible.

Experimentally, the two-step "hypothesis" does not appear to be generally valid.

HOST FACTORS IN TUMOR INDUCTION

Small causes can have extensive effects. In Newton's mechanics this is not the case; there, for every force there corresponds an opposing force, for every *action* an equal and opposite *reaction.*

In complicated regulatory systems, however, even very small regulatory forces can evoke very large effects. The simple example of turning on a faucet demonstrates the disproportionate relationship between regulatory energy (of the hand) and useful work (of the water works). Even someone who knows all there is to know about an ignition key need not have any idea of the mechanisms which result in the motion of his automobile. Similarly, even someone who understands the chemistry of carcinogens in detail still does not know very much about the processes set in motion by these substances. Thus, in this situation, too, as so often otherwise, a simple cause-and-effect relationship is replaced by *uncoupling causality*. In such systems, even the most intimate knowledge of the uncoupling agent says absolutely nothing about what is triggered.

Small changes in a molecule can lead to dramatic changes in its biological properties (Figure 14). Androgens and estrogens, male and female hormones, are quite similar in their basic skeletons. Both are steroids, with four carbon rings fused together. Yet their effects are entirely different, such that isolated effects lead from trivial metabolic interactions to morphological changes and finally to psychic variations.

Viruses offer particularly impressive examples for the dependance of biological properties on chemical fine structure. For example, if a

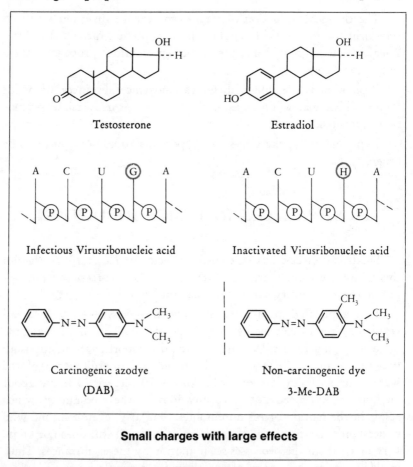

Testosterone

Estradiol

Infectious Virusribonucleic acid

Inactivated Virusribonucleic acid

Carcinogenic azodye

(DAB)

Non-carcinogenic dye

3-Me-DAB

Small charges with large effects

Figure 14

healthy tobacco plant is treated with a ribonucleic acid preparation from tobacco mosaic virus, after a few days the first signs of serious disease appear; soon the leaves wither and the plant dies. Now, a similar virus RNA preparation which has had a change (on the average) in only one out of every 2,000 building blocks is without effect. The plants remain healthy, as if nothing had happened. Such minimal changes can be effected, for example, with sodium nitrite, in that nothing but an exchange of an amino group for a hydroxy group in a guanine or adenine residue takes place. The remainder of the molecule is unchanged. Yet this trivial modification of a single building block in the RNA suffices to make a harmless molecule out of this highly infectious ribonucleic acid.

The differences between carcinogens and noncarcinogens can also be apparently trivial. If mice are painted with a solution of 3,4-benzpyrene, papillomas and carcinomas eventually appear. 1,2-Benzpyrene, on the other hand, causes no tumors during the life time of the animal. Consider another example: N,N-dimethyl-4-aminoazobenzene is carcinogenic, but 2-methyl-DAB is not; the introduction of a single methyl group wipes out carcinogenic activity.

Up to this point we have looked at carcinogenesis primarily from the perspective of chemical carcinogens. It is now necessary to pick up some pieces, to find out what the organism contributes, what factors other than the carcinogen itself control carcinogenesis. A complete description of these factors is still impossible, so let us be content with a few examples. Consider first the barriers raised against a carcinogen which is to induce a tumor.

The Path to the Inner Sanctum

The first problem for a carcinogen is to get into a cell; but cells are exclusive, and their membranes are very picky about which substances in what quantities are admitted from the environment (Figure 15). Cell membranes consist primarily of lipophilic building blocks, and this situation alone effects a certain limitation on transport into the cell. A purely fat-soluble substance will get stuck in the membranes, for it will be most difficult for it to cross intervening aqueous regions. Conversely, a primarily water-soluble compound will hardly be able to push through lipid-containing membranes, but will be repulsed as a drop of water from an oily surface.

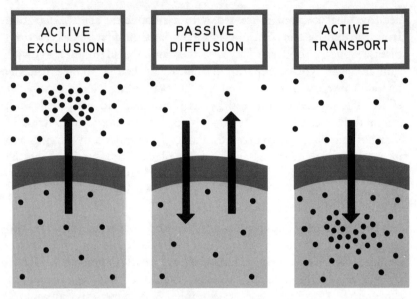

Figure 15

The relative solubility of a substance in hydrophilic and hydrophobic solvents can be measured quantitatively. In this technique the substance in question is "partitioned" between immiscible aqueous and nonaqueous solvents, and its concentration in the two liquids is then measured. Hansch and Fujita have partitioned a series of compounds derived in common manner from carcinogenic and noncarcinogenic azo dyes. Using n-octanol and water as the two liquids, they obtained a remarkable correlation between the "partition coefficients" of these compounds and carcinogenic activities. High water solubility and also high fat solubility indicated reduced carcinogenicity. There were exceptions, to be sure, but this should not be surprising, for cell membranes are certainly more than simply passive barriers which protect the inside of the cell from certain substances.

It has been shown time and again that living cells are in a position to actively take in certain compounds. In a few cases people have analyzed more closely the "permeases" (operationally, still only "mechanisms" which permit permeation against a concentration gradient necessary for such an operation). Permeases for carcinogenic compounds have not yet been described, but their existence must be taken into consideration.

Possibly the problem for a carcinogen is not to get into a cell, but to keep from getting thrown out again. Protective mechanisms which permit a cell to free itself of unwanted substances could also be dangerous to carcinogens, but here, too, there is no experimental proof. Only for cortisol is there probable evidence that L-cells can push out cortisol that has once forced its way in. This evidence consists of the observation that, if the energy production of L-cells is blocked, they take up *more* cortisol than do L-cells in normal circumstances.

Thus, the path of a carcinogen in a cell probably does not depend alone on its solubility properties. Still, there are even more reasons why Hansch had to find exceptions.

Activation of Carcinogens as a Limiting Step in Chemical Carcinogenesis

Even if a carcinogen succeeds in being taken up by a cell, this is a long way from ensuring that carcinogenesis begins. Many carcinogens must first be converted to the actual active forms via cell metabolism, and here there are differences among cells. Some cells can activate, some cannot. At least, this is the opinion of many authors when it comes to explaining why certain carcinogens selectively induce tumors in certain organs and tissues. (This selectivity toward certain cells has occasionally been called organotropy.)

Now because (in general) carcinogens must be activated, it is important how and especially where a carcinogen is applied. Take an example from skin carcinogenesis to illustrate: if acetylaminofluorene (AAF) is applied directly to the skin of a mouse, later treatment with croton oil is ineffective in inducing papillomas. In contrast, this combination works quite well if AAF is fed instead of "painted." Activated AAF derivatives can then reach the skin after first arising in the liver. We have already seen what such an activation might look like:

$$Ar-N\genfrac{}{}{0pt}{}{\diagup COCH_3}{\diagdown H} \xrightarrow{O_2} Ar-N\genfrac{}{}{0pt}{}{\diagup COCH_3}{\diagdown OH} \longrightarrow Ar-N\genfrac{}{}{0pt}{}{\diagup COCH_3}{\diagdown OCOCH_3}$$

Nitrosamines are also converted to reactive intermediates in cellular metabolism, with oxidation playing a decisive role here too:

$$ON-N\begin{matrix}CH_3\\\\CH_3\end{matrix}\xrightarrow[TPNH]{O_2}ON-N\begin{matrix}CH_2OH\\\\CH_3\end{matrix}\longrightarrow[CH_3{}^+]$$

Dimethylnitrosamine

For the closely related nitrosamides (for example, nitrosomethylurea), however, there is obviously no activation necessary. Simple hydrolysis suffices to lead to reactive end products:

$$O=C\begin{matrix}NH_2\\\\CH_3\\N\\\\NO\end{matrix}\xrightarrow{H_2O}[CH_3-\underset{H}{N}-NO]\longrightarrow[CH_3{}^+]$$

Such carcinogens which can do without activation and which do not pick up their disruptive properties in metabolism might be exceptional.

Occasionally the activating reactions are referred to as *toxication*, for it is only in the organism that the actual toxins are produced. The opposite of these processes are the much better known *detoxication* reactions. These, too, play an important role in carcinogenesis: they are processes which the carcinogens must avoid. Obviously, toxication and detoxication are anthropomorphic concepts, since in reality they are only two sides of the same coin.

Danger for Carcinogens: Detoxication Reactions

If one feeds carcinogenic hydrocarbons such as 3,4-benzpyrene or 3-methylcholanthrene to a mouse or a rat, these animals excrete a multitude of changed hydrocarbons. Often it is simply a matter of introduction of oxygen (hydroxylation). Some of these hydroxylated hydrocarbons have been prepared in "large" quantities and tested for carcinogenic activity, always with the same result: these derivatives of highly active carcinogens are completely inactive.

The conclusion that these are in fact detoxication products is not at all certain. If hydroxylated carcinogenic hydrocarbons can pass cell membranes only with difficulty — possibly because they are then more water soluble — then they would not serve as carcinogens, even if they should be carcinogenic once inside the cell. Thus, the direct test for carcinogenicity cannot always give clear results.

Reactivation of Glucuronides in the Urine: Bladder Cancer

Activated carcinogens can be converted to ethers (glycosides) of glucuronic acid:

They are then excreted by the kidney through the ureter to the urinary bladder. But here their carcinogenic effects can flare up once more; urine contains glucuronidase, an enzyme that can set these carcinogens free once more.

This mechanism appears to be significant in the appearance of bladder cancer resulting from aromatic amines: man and the dog possess this glucuronidase; mice and rats do not. It follows naturally that man and dogs are susceptible to these tumors and that mice and rats are not.

Thus, the production of bladder tumors by aromatic amines is determined by an alternation between activating, deactivating, and reactivating reactions. More simply, the "strength" of an applied carcinogen, as well as the site of tumor induction, depends considerably on the metabolism of these substances.

All the processes with which we have become acquainted are decisive in the question of whether a tumor can occur or not. Central to this question are the carcinogens themselves, their permeation through cell membranes, their activation in metabolism, and their detoxication. Still, a carcinogen must not only find a suitable cell, it must find it at the appropriate moment.

Phase Rule of Carcinogenesis

A single meal (of carcinogen) can be sufficient to induce mammary cancer. Huggins was able to induce mammary gland carcinomas in 100 percent of female Sprague-Dawley rats by a single intubation of methylcholanthrene or DMBA (100 or 20 mg/rat, respectively) in sesame oil at 50–65 days of age. Feeding at either an earlier or later time point drastically reduced the tumor yields. Thus, the correct age of the animal decides the success or failure of the experiment; obviously the mammary gland cells are in an especially sensitive phase between 50 and 65 days.

Naturally, we must take into account indirect effects. Mammary gland cells especially are hormone-dependent, and it is entirely possible that the special sensitivity depends on an especially favorable hormonal pattern. Such indirect effects are excluded in in vitro experiments, yet it has turned out that for "carcinogenesis in a test tube" it is also important to catch the cells in the correct phase (see page 200).

Thus, if all the "switches" have been set correctly, we get formation of a tumor cell. Getting to a full-grown tumor is farther down the line, however.

Tumor Cells can be Dormant

Clinicians repeatedly are confronted with the disappointing experience of seeing patients develop the same tumors, often at other locations, decades after apparently successful surgical excision — so-called late metastases. For example, after surgical removal of a primary breast carcinoma, metastases can appear in a lumbar vertebra 25–30 years later. Such cases demonstrate that cancer cells "literally are able to lead a dormant existence in the organism for years and decades" (K. H. Bauer).

Not only migratory tumor cells are dormant. Occasionally tumor cells remain "frozen in" at the site of their induction. Numerous clinical examples are also available to demonstrate this possibility, for example, the so-called carcinoma in situ, malignant tumors before the catastrophic take-off. These are frequently diagnosed in skin, in the larynx, in breast tissue, but especially in the uterine cervix (see Figure 54). Particularly in the case of cervical carcinoma in situ, considerable quantities of cells with unambiguous neoplastic character can be formed which do not, however, break through the basal membrane, which separates the epithelium from the tissue underneath. The cell masses sit there clearly separated from the lower layers of tissue and have not begun invasive growth. Minor surgery — assuming early diagnosis — permits complete cure at this stage. In spite of the significance of carcinoma in situ for medicine, suitable models for it do not exist for animal experiments.

Still, proof of existence of latent tumor cells in rats and hamsters has been obtained. Fisher and Fisher injected 50 Walker carcinoma cells into the portal veins of rats. After many months, no tumors had appeared either in the liver or anywhere else. On the other hand, if other similarly treated rats were laparotomized several times in the interval (simple surgical opening and closing of the peritoneal cavity and manipulation of the liver), Walker carcinomas were found in the livers. This experiment shows that latent Walker cells did exist in the liver and that they could be awakened by simple traumatic processes.

Paradoxical Influences of Nutrition

As a general rule, life is more difficult for tumor cells in an undernourished host (Tannenbaum). Boutwell, among others, has conducted experiments in skin carcinogenesis under dietary deficiency. When his mice received only 60 percent of the amount of food that they would have eaten ad libitum, then the number of animals with papillomas (after 16 weeks of promotion with croton oil) was reduced from the control value of 50 percent down to merely 14 percent, and the average number of papillomas per mouse fell from 6 to less than 2.

Bullough has proposed an explanation dear to his own heart: undernourished animals live under constant stress, which means that stress hormones, such as adrenalin and cortisone, are at a constant elevated level. It is known that these hormones particularly can inhibit mitoses. In this way the inhibition of tumor yields is simply explained. In any case, cortisone itself has the expected effect on tumor yields. In an initiation-promotion experiment, the administration of 0.5 mg of cortisone/mouse per day in the diet reduced the number of animals with carcinomas to 10 percent of the control value (Boutwell). Still dietary deficiency does not always aid tumor suppression: DAB hepatomas, for example, can be induced only if the rats are maintained on a protein-deficient diet. A complete protein diet protects against tumor induction in this case.

One other curiosity probably deserves mention: choline deficiency alone is sufficient to induce hepatomas in rats.

Hormone-Dependent Tumor Growth

Many tumors are dependent on hormones. Foulds observed a particularly dramatic example in mice: spontaneous mammary carcinomas grew rapidly during a pregnancy. After birth, their growth slowed or even regressed. At the next pregnancy there was a new wave of growth. In this case, therefore, tumor growth depends quite clearly on hormonal patterns. The mammary carcinomas, at least at first, are "hormone dependent." In the course of their further development, however, these mouse carcinomas lost their dependency and grew without further pregnancies until the animals eventually died.

Mammary gland carcinomas in rats are essentially always hormone dependent. A simple experiment demonstrates this dependency: breast cancer in rats regresses after surgical removal of the ovaries. The "cocarcinogenic" effect of female sex hormones is even necessary for virus-induced mammary cancer; we will come back later to the example of the Bittner-Virus in the Virus chapter (page 152).

Sometimes, however, the removal of sex glands can occasion malignant growth. Experienced hunters are acquainted with the situation of bucks with malformed antlers in which bone grows incessantly and without assuming the characteristic normal forms, eventually killing the animal. These hunters also know the cause of these malignant formations: the buck had previously suffered damage to the scrotum. Such a case, to be sure, is a rare curiosity for the hunter's trophy case, but it, too, demonstrates the significance of a balanced hormonal budget for growth regulation.

Besides the sex hormones, the pituitary is decisive in tumor growth. Instead of removing the ovaries, one can extirpate the pituitary in order to stop mammary carcinomas. Conversely, mammary carcinomas can be experimentally induced by implanting a second pituitary in a mouse. This supplementary pituitary can be introduced under the skin, into the spleen, or even under the renal capsule: in each case the excessive supply of pituitary hormone leads to neoplastic growth.

Breast tissue is also normally dependent on (female sexual) hormones; a dependence of the tumor tissue derived from it is therefore highly plausible. Yet even in organs which normally are not targets for hormones, hormonal effects can be important for carcinogenesis. Reuber found that hepatomas can be induced by AAF only in the presence of thyroxine and testosterone. The two hormones can be cut off by thyroidectomy and castration, respectively: after this double operation, liver tumors fail to occur. Supplementary dosing with thyroxine and testosterone again permits induction of hepato-cellular carcinomas (Figure 16).

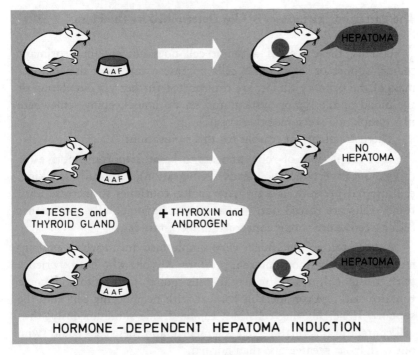

Figure 16

The influence of hormones on tumor induction and tumor growth is peculiar to each tumor to a high degree. All of the peculiarities are not known, but that tumor growth can be influenced by hormones has been known for more than a century. As early as 1836, Cooper established a connection between breast carcinomas and menstruation.

Tumor Cells Must Slip Past the Immune Response

Our knowledge about the influence of the host's immune system on tumor growth is much more recent. This system, with its antibody-producing cells and active lymphocytes which can kill foreign cells directly, registers everything "foreign" in an organism: bacteria and viruses are foreign, and the entire arsenal of antibodies is disposable against them. Obviously, tumor cells which have arisen from the normal cells of a tissue are also foreign. Thus, this defense specific to the host is a basic danger for all tumor cells (see pp. 124 ff.).

The Pattern of Metastases is Also Determined by the Host

Usually the career of a tumor cell does not end in a primary tumor. Sooner or later tumor cells migrate away from the compact mass of the primary tumor, are transported further via circulation of the blood or the lymph system, and set up housekeeping somewhere in a lymph node or some other tissue.

There are plenty of reasons for this emigration:

1. A simple lack of room appears to be an important motive for this exodus (overpopulation leads to emigration). Physically speaking, the internal pressure in a primary tumor continues to increase until tumor cells are forced out. Measurements have actually shown that such excessive pressure is concerned in metastasizing.

2. Leighton pointed out a very simple mechanism which explains metastasis even without internal pressure. Anyone who has experience with tissue cultures knows that cells going into mitosis become rounded and lose considerable contact with neighboring cells and the support. If neighboring cells in a tumor divide simultaneously, then cell contact in this small region is loosened, and these cells could swim out with much greater ease than normal.

3. As formulated by Foulds, tumor cells have a life history, in which they develop more and more in the direction of autonomy. Foulds coined the concept of progression for this situation: "The basic idea of progression is the same as that of epigenetic development in embryology." Invasive growth and metastasizing growth are stations in this progression; a prerequisite for both is the loss of neighborly relationships.

Obviously, when and if a tumor metastasizes depends on the tumor cells themselves and on their immediate surroundings. The host, however, has an important word to put in about where the ejected cells migrate, where they settle down, and where they blossom out to daughter tumors.

It has long been noteworthy to clinicians and experimental oncologists that metastases normally are not spread evenly through the organism, but appear preferentially in certain tissues. The spleen, for example, is almost always spared, while the liver, lungs, and lymph nodes are favorite targets. The affection of certain tumor cells for certain organs can reach extreme degrees: for example, Kinsey found a mouse melanoma (S-91) with a special affinity for lung tissue. If this melanoma was inoculated into mice with lung tissue implanted in the leg, the melanoma grew only in lung tissue, all right, but in the implanted pieces of lung as well as in the normal lung.

Experiments of this type led to the supposition that certain tissues represent an especially "congenial soil" for certain tumor cells. Still, this idea might not suffice to explain all patterns of metastases. Foulds suggested, for example, "that some organs, notably the spleen, resist the establishment of secondary deposits by a local mechanism similar to that which opposes the takes of grafts in laboratory animals." Finally, simple hemodynamic effects could considerably influence the transport and deposit of migrating tumor cells. Only in those places to which tumor cells really have access, where they can "hang around," can metastases be formed at all (Walther). To be sure, many investigations have shown that the purely mechanical distribution of tumor cells throughout the entire organism is not a problem.

Schmähl and Riesenberg, for example, injected intravenously high cell counts of a transplantable ascites tumor, which grows in the lung after this method of administration. They killed the animals after certain times, prepared cell breis from the different organs, and injected them separately into healthy rats intraperitoneally. The "taking" of an ascites tumor would then prove the presence of tumor cells in the respective brei. In this manner, 1 hour after intravenous injection of Walker tumor cells, viable tumor cells could be demonstrated in all of the investigated organs (lung, liver, kidney, spleen, and whole blood). After 24 hours, only the lung preparation yielded tumor-inducing material. From this we can conclude that there is hardly any hindrance to the distribution of tumor cells and that many organs initially "sown" with tumor cells contain no more viable cells after a certain period. The argument that the lung is the first filter in this experiment does not hold water, since other tumors in the same protocol "metastasize" according to completely different distribution patterns.

"There now seems to be a general feeling that the congenial soil theory and the mechanicocirculatory theory should not be thought of as conflicting and mutually exclusive, but as complementary" (Leighton).

Summary: Host Factors, or the "Game Plan" of Tumor Development

Chemical carcinogenesis is a pathway with roadblocks: at many points on this pathway there can be a decision as to whether the final effect will be a tumor cell or not. There are difficulties in forcing entry into the cell, in activation to the actual active form, and in detoxication of the carcinogens. Only when sufficient carcinogen enters a cell, only when it is converted to reactive products, and if it is not again inactivated by detoxifying enzymes, then, and only then, does a carcinogen have a chance to transform a cell. "Carcinogens must fit in many keyholes."

They must not only fit, they have to turn the lock at the right moment. Whether a neoplastic transformation takes place or not obviously may depend on that stage of the cell cycle in which a carcinogen attacks a cell.

All of these decisions taken together contribute to the more or less selective conversion of certain cell types to tumor cells by certain carcinogens. The expression *organotropy* has been coined for this selective sensitivity.

Even finished tumor cells are not out of the woods. They must avoid the immune defense system of the host, and as a rule they are made aware that certain hormones are at their disposal. In the example of the mouse mammary carcinoma studied by Foulds, it became clear how much changing "hormone fields" can influence changes in tumor growth. The immune response and hormone level are only two examples of many possible regulatory fields of the organism with which the tumor cell must reckon. The regulatory fields of a tissue itself are primarily important for the survival of a tumor cell. We have not mentioned tissue-specific regulatory possibilities, but it is just these which might play a highly decisive role in carcinogenesis. Consequently, we will take up this subject in more detail in the next chapter.

Even in the last lap of the natural history of a tumor cell, at the progression into metastasis, the tumor cell is dependent on the host organism. Hemodynamic factors together with "biochemical" peculiarities determine the target tissue of the settling pattern.

Finally, simple changes in the host's nutrition can influence tumor development. DAB hepatomas can be induced only with protein-deficient diets. Low calorie diets, on the other hand, inhibit carcinoma formation in skin (Tannenbaum).

In the chess game "carcinogen vs. cell," only a few moves are correct. The carcinogen is playing not only against the target cell, but against the entire organism.

TISSUE-SPECIFIC GROWTH REGULATION ("CHALONES")

The size of an organism is by no means determined by pure chance: "Man, as a lung-using animal, cannot be as small as an insect, and vice versa. Only occasionally, as in the case of the Goliath beetle, do the sizes of beetles and mice meet and overlap. Thus, each group of animals has its upper and lower limits" (D'Arcy Thompson).

Simple physical laws appear to establish these limits: warm-blooded animals must balance their heat loss by constant heat production. Heat radiation is proportioned to surface area, but heat production is proportional to weight. Consequently, a smaller animal must produce more heat (relative to its size) than a larger, and consequently smaller animals require more nutrition: a man consumes daily about one-fiftieth of his body weight in food, but in two days a mouse eats its entire weight in food. Thus, warmblooded animals much smaller than mice are "forbidden."

In insects, the unique respiratory system sets a limit to growth in size: the trachea supply oxygen to the insect's body directly, but simple diffusion in this simple plumbing system functions without complications only on a small scale.

Even if we know why a mouse can be no smaller than it is, we are still far from knowing why it, or a rat, or a rabbit, attains only a certain size from which it deviates only slightly in normal situations. Certainly individual size is determined by heredity and environment, but this says nothing about which factors, which forces, really limit growth.

Even the single organs of an organism are subject to strict growth limitations; for here, too, there are "invisible boundaries," beyond which growth is not permitted. These invisible boundaries are especially impressive in the case of liver regeneration: if one removes two-thirds of a rat's liver, the remainder grows back to a normal liver within a short time. This vehement growth is abruptly braked, however, as soon as the original size is again attained.

Hence, the size of an organ, too, is by no means determined by simple chance. The question then arises, which regulatory forces are active here. Indirect mechanisms, such as nerve stimulation or even hormonal alterations, certainly are involved, but the decisive regulatory impulses might emanate from the tissue itself. Therefore, we are going to examine the "regulatory field" of the tissue somewhat more closely, for this "field" appears to pay an important role in carcinogenesis.

Cybernetic Model of Tissue-Specific Growth Regulation

How does technology solve the problem (as an example) of maintaining a constant fluid level? Even with a simple set-up a constant loss from a vessel (possibly by evaporation) can be compensated for automatically (Figure 17). A balance must indicate the deviation from the desired value, with this deviation coupled to a valve which regulates addition of liquid from a supply vessel. When the desired value of liquid quantity is obtained, the valve is closed and further addition of liquid is stopped (principle of negative feedback).

P. Weiss has developed a model for (liver) regeneration using this same principle. The premise of the Weiss model is simple: single cells of a tissue produce an inhibitor which blocks division of just those cells. Liver parenchymal cells produce inhibitors for liver parenchymal cells, "skin cells" for skin cells and so forth. Many cells inhibit strongly, a few only weakly (see page 219). Using this proposition, we can understand how, in liver regeneration,

1. cell division first increases, and
2. why a cessation of growth takes place after completed regeneration.

This simple picture immediately runs up against difficulties: thus, "strict" theory distinguishes between cells which produce inhibitor

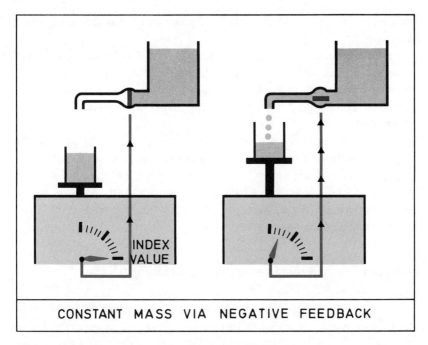

CONSTANT MASS VIA NEGATIVE FEEDBACK

Figure 17

and those which react to it. With this model one can avoid the dilemma of requiring that inhibitor-producing cells not react themselves to the inhibitors.

This "cybernetic theory" of liver regeneration predicts the existences of diffusible inhibitors to be found between liver cells or possibly in the circulatory system of the whole organism ("humoral inhibitors").

Regulation of Liver Regeneration by Humoral Inhibitors

"The literature on liver regeneration is large and contradictory, mainly because so much of the experimental work was inadequately planned. In fact, the only conclusion which seems to be generally accepted is that the message to commence regeneration must be humoral" (Bullough).

This conclusion is supported by two experiments:

1. Two rats can be surgically connected, in the manner of Siamese twins, so that their vascular systems grow together (parabiosis). If part of the liver in *one* of the rats is removed, an increase in mitoses in *both* livers is observed. The common circulation supplies informa-

tion about the state of the operated liver over into the unoperated animal.

2. In a similar experiment, an extra piece of liver was transplanted into an "abnormal" spot in a rat. Partial hepatectomy was then performed on the rat, and here, too, both liver tissues, the residual normal liver and the transplanted piece of tissue, responded with a wave of mitoses.

These two experiments show that signaling substances exist in the blood; exactly this finding was predicted by cybernetic theory. Bullough has coined the name "chalone" for such a substance. The most important findings on the existence, properties, and mode of action of these chalones were obtained not with liver, but with skin. Thus, we must again turn to the latter tissue.

Skin as a Regenerating System ("Wound Healing")

Even under normal conditions a continuous regeneration of skin is taking place; the uppermost horny layer is constantly being sloughed off, and continuous replacement from the lower cell layers accompanies this process. The total period for replacement of the entire epidermis amounts to barely a week in the mouse.

The *vis regenerativa* of the epidermis is primarily revealed at times of minor mechanical destruction; within a few days the original condition is reestablished. (It is only in the case of major injury that scar tissue forms from connective tissue cells.)

Here, too, the "chalone theory" offers a plausible interpretation: because of the loss of the chalone-producing skin cells, the chalone concentration falls in the cells neighboring the wound. But a reduced level of inhibitor means cell division.

First Bullough, then Iversen, made the following test of this idea; if chalones really exist, then it should be possible to extract them from skin cells. Upon injection of a simple aqueous extract, the number of mitoses in the skin could actually be reduced by half, without influencing the mitoses in the liver or other organs.

Bullough investigated the effect of chalone-containing extracts, especially in vitro, on small pieces of mouse ear, but here the simple skin extracts did not have the expected effect. Success was obtained only upon addition of certain hormones, but to appreciate this we have to introduce some more background.

Stress Hormones Suppress Mitoses

It has long been known that, in the tissues of adult mammals, the number of mitoses follows a daily rhythm. In the epidermis more cells divide when the animal is sleeping than when it is awake.

The variation in adrenalin level is shifted in phase from the above rhythm: in the active animal it is at a high level; it is low in the resting animal. Bullough found that there is an exactly inverse proportion between the mitotic activity of the epidermis and the adrenalin level in the blood. Adrenalin injections or stress situations, which accelerate adrenalin excretion, lead as expected to mitotic inhibition. Another stress hormone, hydrocortisone, similarly proved to be antimitotic. With adrenalin and hydrocortisone, chalone effects could then be demonstrated in vitro (Bullough).

Epidermal Chalone in an in vitro Experiment

A typical in vitro preparation contains pieces of skin in 4 ml of nutrient medium (glucose/salts/buffer) together with skin extract and 10 µg each of adrenalin and hydrocortisone. Mitosis is arrested by addition of colchicine, and after 4 hours the experiment is stopped. The pieces of skin are fixed, stained, and the mitoses counted. Under suitable conditions, the addition of skin extract reduces the number of mitoses by half; the hormones adrenalin and hydrocortisone are indispensable as "coinhibitors."

Colchicine has nothing to do with the actual experiment; it arrests mitoses and thus simply facilitates counting. All mitoses that occur during the time period of the experiment can be counted together at the end.

Similarly prepared extracts from other organs were without effect on skin pieces; conversely, skin extracts did nothing to explants of liver and other organs. Accordingly, the chalone effect is *organ specific*.

Mitoses in mouse ear can be effectively blocked not only with mouse skin extracts, but also with preparations from codfish skin, pigskin, or even human skin. Chalones obviously are *not species specific*.

Tentative Characterization of the Epidermal Chalone

Large quantities of pigskin accumulate in the abattoirs of the pharmaceutical concern, Organon. In cooperation with Bullough, the biochemical research laboratories of this firm were thus consequently able to extract rather large quantities of epidermal pigskin chalone. Alcohol precipitations between 60 and 80 percent along with electrophoresis led to an enrichment of about 2,000-fold. Analyses showed that a protein was involved, possibly a glycoprotein. Sedimentation in the analytical ultracentrifuge indicated a molecular weight between 30,000 and 40,000 (Hondius-Bolding).

Chalones can Block Mitosis Directly

Why do chalones inhibit? How does this mitosis brake function? Let us again consider skin cells, in particular the basal cells of the epidermis. The cells of this cell state form the reservoir for the cells lying above them, the so-called differentiated keratin-producing cells, which finally make up the uppermost horny layer.

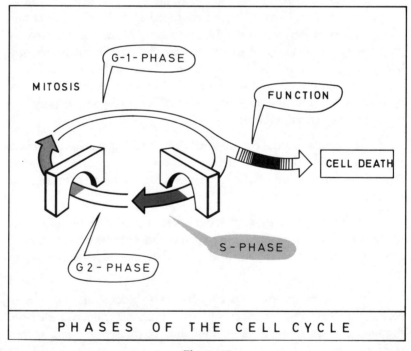

Figure 18

The life history of these cells can be divided up according to the terminology of the cytologists. After a phase in which DNA is synthesized (S-phase), there comes an intermediate phase (G-2) followed by mitosis. A G-1 phase then completes the cell cycle. (Cells that no longer divide can branch off into a "function phase.") The question is, then: do chalones block the S-phase or mitosis, i. e., do they slam a door to entrance into mitosis or before entrance into DNA synthesis?

Already after 4 hours, Bullough observed a dramatic effect on the number of mitoses. Since the cell phases (S and G-2) coming before mitosis require more than 4 hours, the chalones do in fact close the door on mitosis directly. With this, however, the story begins to have problems: in a tissue in which the cells can replicate their DNA and are braked just before mitosis, there would have to be many cells with double the normal DNA content (so-called 4n cells). In many tissues, and unfortunately in epidermis too, this is not the case. Hence, a second brake would have to be postulated, which can take effect even before the S-phase. Newer investigations have in fact shown that there are not only tissue-specific inhibitors which block mitosis, but also some which close the door before the S-phase (Elgjö, Marks). These inhibitors would be the "true" chalones.

Alternatives to the Chalone Theory: Wound Hormones

The chalone theory is not the only theory invented to explain regeneration. The most important competitor is the "wound hormone." According to this concept, the cells themselves of an injured tissue produce stimulating factors. Cells, according to this theory, "hibernate"; additional stimulation reawakens them. These alarms were and still are sought under the name wound hormones. However, we lack convincing reports of success. "In spite of more than 50 years of effort, all such substances remain hypothetical, and until one of them has been extracted and characterized it remains reasonable to question their reality" (Bullough). Success in this objective has in fact been achieved with tissue-specific inhibitors. Therefore, we will examine the "chalone concept" more closely.

Chalones as Repressors

In order to set a pendulum in motion, there are two possibilities open:

1. strike it directly ("wound hormone") or
2. release a raised pendulum ("chalone concept").

"Stimulation" or "removal of an inhibition" have the same effect, but their mechanisms are basically different. In the one case, the cells must be excited into division; in the other, it is sufficient to release a brake — the cells can then take off by themselves.

Embryonic development seems to make a case for a braking effect: cells of a tissue divide during development, and it as clear that these divisions are then braked to a halt at the end of development.

This same problem, stimulation vs. removal of an inhibition, has already been thoroughly discussed, in the matter of enzyme induction in bacteria. *E. coli* grow normally with glucose as their carbon source. It is possible, however, to culture them on media containing lactose as the sugar, but then the bacteria must first synthesize specific enzymes with which they can "digest" the lactose (galactosidase). The induction of these enzymes by lactose in the medium makes growth possible for the bacteria even under abnormal conditions.

Previously it was assumed that the cells "learned" to make galactosidase only after contact with the lactose. According to our present concepts, an *E. coli* cell "knows" from the first how to make galactosidase. This knowledge is brought into play, however, only when it is really needed, that is, when the cell is forced to make use of lactose. If there is no lactose present, then no lactose-cleaving enzyme is produced, for reasons of economy.

We cannot discuss the details of how this enzyme induction goes on. The result of many experiments and considerations is the following scheme (the Jacob-Monod model):

A specific galactosidase repressor normally inhibits the activity of the galactosidase gene, which represents the blueprint for these enzymes ("structural gene"). To this end the repressor must react with an "operator gene" adjacent to the structural gene. If the cell now comes in contact with lactose, the galactosidase repressor reacts with this sugar and is removed from the scene. It can no longer cover up the operator, and the structural gene can now produce enzyme.

The induction of enzymes is thus not induction via a template substrate, but removal of an inhibition, which previously had hindered the synthesis of unnecessary enzymes.

Now, the same scheme that holds for bacterial enzyme induction can also be carried over into the chalone theory (Figure 19). The chalone corresponds to the repressor; however, it does not simply

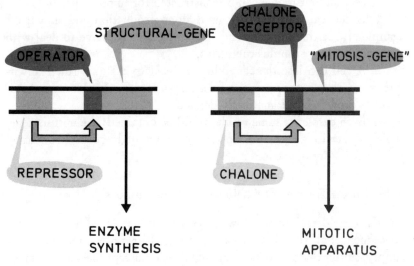

Figure 19

repress a single certain gene, but an entire gene complex. This complex encompasses all genes necessary for conducting mitosis. The locus of the mitosis gene complex to which the chalone attaches is usually known as the chalone receptor; it would correspond to the classical operator.

The question is still open as to whether chalones attach directly to this receptor or whether they indirectly release substances which in turn occupy the receptor. There is often thought to be a primary reaction between chalone and cell membrane, but for our further discussion it is unimportant whether chalones act at the gene level or at the level of the membrane.

Tumor Cells as Chalone Mutants

Bacterial cells can forget to "think" economically: even without necessity, they then produce — occasionally in tremendous quantities — unnecessary galactosidase. This enzyme then also constitutes part of the standard enzyme equipment of these mutants ("constitutive mutants"). The Jacob-Monod model offers two possibilities to explain the occurrence of such a constitutive mutant — either the repressor or the operator is damaged. In both cases an effective blockade of the structural gene is no longer possible: even without substrate inactivation of the repressor, enzyme synthesis takes place.

A very similar model can be constructed for tumor cells:

1. A cell can throttle back its chalone production and shut it off completely. A chalone deficiency develops, and we have to deal with a supplementary stimulus to mitosis.

2. A cell can lose the capability to react to chalones (their antennae for chalones, the receptors, are out of order). In this case, autonomous growth is automatically defined.

In both cases, the same result would be obtained: the mitosis gene, which otherwise goes into action strictly regulated, would be switched onto continuous operation.

Substitution Therapy of Chalone-Deficient Tumors

The considerations which we have already advanced have a simple consequence: all tumors that have not lost their chalone receptors and simply suffer chalone deficiency should be susceptible to treatment with supplemental chalone.

There appear to be such tumors: Bullough discovered an epidermal epithelial carcinoma which can be inhibited by epidermal chalone — skin powder. This is the so-called VX-tumor of the rabbit, a transplantable tumor originally induced by the Shope virus. Pig skin extracts served as a source of chalone.

What Bullough could show, to be sure, were only in vitro effects: skin powder choked off the mitotic counts in tumor slices. For an in vivo "cure" there was simply not enough material available for the rabbit, despite mass production from pig skin. Still, the VX-tumor was not an isolated case; Rytömaa found a chalone-sensitive chloroleukemia, and Mohr successfully treated hamster and mouse melanomas with skin powder.

The effect of pig skin powder on melanomas was actually discovered by accident: Mohr had attempted with these preparations primarily to influence skin carcinomas induced by carcinogens. In these experiments the subcutaneously transplanted melanomas were intended to serve as negative controls, but the results were the exact reverse: the skin carcinomas remained unaffected — except for an observable wound cleaning — and the melanomas regressed. They became black, softened, and were absorbed or broke through the skin. After the initial astonishment, these findings were also fitted into the "chalone concept": skin, pig skin included, contains normal melanocytes, which on work-up are naturally also extracted. But normal melanocytes contain "melanocyte chalone" — and this in turn inhibits melanoma cells.

Bullough was not the first to attack tumors with organ extracts. A gigantic literature describes earlier successful and unsuccessful attempts. Now the chalone theory has given the "alchemy of organ extracts" a rational background, and the Bullough in vitro systems made exact experiments possible for the first time. On the other hand, the real possibility of using chalones in therapy of spontaneous tumors seems highly doubtful.

Chalones, a General Principle?

"Chalone research" has won many new friends because of the possible application, however doubtful, in a "physiological tumor therapy." Kidney chalones, lung chalones, and uterus chalones have been announced. However, the carelessness with which extractions and applications have often been done makes it difficult to believe in a general principle. Further developments must be awaited; above all it is essential that we not settle into too narrow a view: besides negative growth regulators, positive regulators are still very probably part of the picture. Many growth-stimulating substances have been described; the best known is now the nerve growth factor, but an epithelial growth factor — from the salivary glands of mice — has been isolated and purified (Cohen). Why shouldn't physiological growth regulation also rest on an interplay between stimulating and inhibitory impulses?

"Visible" Regulation Fields

In an elegant, extremely simple experiment, Fujii and Mizuno were able to show that signals are exchanged between cells of the epidermis. They implanted small pieces of membrane filter into the epidermis and thus separated the epidermal cells from each other (Figure 20). If they used paraffin-dipped, water-impermeable filters, then the cells grew around the implanted filter until there was again cell contact. The cells could not "hear" through the filter the fact that they had neighbors. In contrast, permeable membranes obviously permitted some signal to pass: the cells did not grow around the implant. Epidermis cells that had previously come in contact with a carcinogen behaved differently, however. Even with permeable mem-

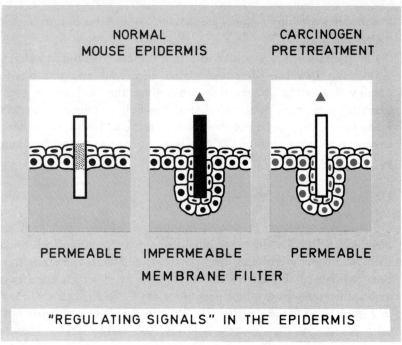

NORMAL MOUSE EPIDERMIS

CARCINOGEN PRETREATMENT

PERMEABLE   IMPERMEABLE   PERMEABLE

MEMBRANE FILTER

"REGULATING SIGNALS" IN THE EPIDERMIS

Figure 20

branes, there was no signal detection and they grew around the barrier.

A simple interpretation: carcinogen-treated cells send their signals with a decreased field strength, so that an intervening piece of filter suffices to weaken the regulatory field to zero. Another interpretation: the field strength is a strong as usual, but the receivers (the cell membranes?) are no longer capable of responding to it. For a further consideration of this point, see the following chapter, in particular the section on cell membranes.

Summary

Chalone is a new name for an old problem. In the adult organism, the cells of a tissue are subject to strict control of division. In the case of regeneration, division is permitted only in measured amounts; after attainment of the original state, mitoses are again blocked. A cybernetic model of explanation has been developed (P. Weiss): the cells of a tissue can produce inhibitors which in turn act on these cells (the principle of negative feedback).

In liver regeneration, signal substances in the circulation transmit important information for the regeneration. Skin-specific inhibitors can be isolated from skin cells and characterized ("epidermal chalones"). Mitoses in epidermis can be inhibited in vitro with such preparations, although only in the presence of the so-called stress hormones adrenalin and hydrocortisone (Bullough). Thus, Bullough has defined chalones as tissue-specific inhibitors that require adrenalin and hydrocortisone as coinhibitors.

The chalone theory offers models for a tumor cell: a) loss of chalones, b) loss of response toward chalones; both lead to neoplastic growth. Tumor cells that simply have too little chalone at their disposal, but that possess intact receptors, should be inhibited by chalones. Such chalone-dependent tumor systems (VX-tumor of the rabbit, chloroleukemia, melanomas?) seem to have been discovered. Clinically "interesting" tumors, such as hydrocarbon-induced skin carcinomas or a transplantable lung carcinoma, were resistant to epidermal chalone.

Still, one can say quite accurately: "if chalones didn't exist, it would be necessary to invent them." The invention, at least, has been successful without doubt.

CARCINOGENESIS AND CELL ORGANELLES

To the first cytologists, a cell was rather simply constructed: it had an outer membrane and a nucleus. The cell body was filled with protoplasm, a substance neither solid nor liquid, which, however, was evidently chosen to be the bearer of life.

People tried everywhere to ferret out the secret of protoplasm using simple model systems. Bütschli, for example, experimented with artificial colloidal droplets of water, oil of cloves, glycerol, and potash; he squeezed them between microscope slides and cover glasses and observed their "lively movements." Zoology professors were not the only ones to construct protoplasm models; "speculators and philosophers" in many small workrooms attempted to experiment with nature, to excite it into wondrous phenomena — to *tempt* it. The thought that animate and inanimate nature formed a single great unity fascinated professionals and amateurs alike. Consequently, simple models ought to supply the key to the secrets of the cell. But in spite of all these efforts, "protoplasm" remained only a name.

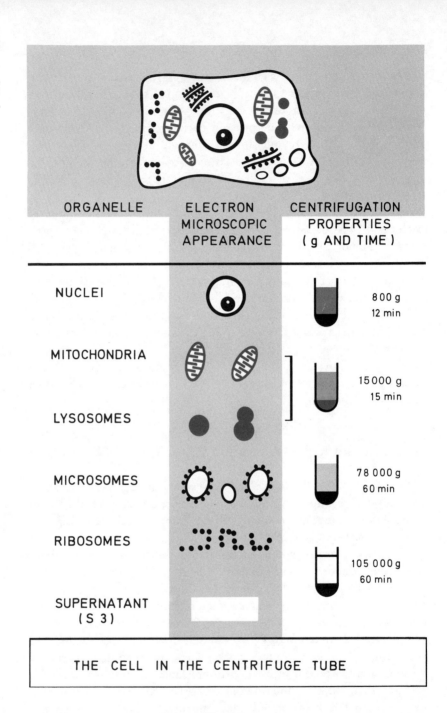

ORGANELLE	ELECTRON MICROSCOPIC APPEARANCE	CENTRIFUGATION PROPERTIES (g AND TIME)
NUCLEI		800 g 12 min
MITOCHONDRIA		15 000 g 15 min
LYSOSOMES		
MICROSOMES		78 000 g 60 min
RIBOSOMES		105 000 g 60 min
SUPERNATANT (S 3)		

THE CELL IN THE CENTRIFUGE TUBE

Figure 21

Today we know that, to be sure, a living cell obeys physical and chemical laws, but that it is impossible to imitate one with simple physicochemical models. The cells of a higher organism are exceedingly complicated structures: besides the nucleus, numerous structures were discovered in the course of time, and even the nucleus could be resolved into different, morphologically definable components.

The Inner Architecture of a Cell

The electron microscope especially gave us important information about the inner structure of a cell (Figure 21). Structures and fine structures that approached molecular dimensions now became visible. (If one were to enlarge the entire animal to a similar extent, to look at it, so to speak, with electron microscopic eyes, one would view rats easily 25 miles long.) The ostensibly homogeneous protoplasm turned out to be a crowded tangle of lamellae, vesicles, particles, and canals. Figure 21 shows in a very schematic manner the most important cell organelles. For reasons of clarity, no attempt was made at a depiction to scale.

Although the electron microscope made visible the inner structures of a cell, it could not, at first, answer the question of which assignments in cell metabolism were given to these structures. The question of function of the cell organelles was first answered with the ultracentrifuge, a machine that enables attainment of acceleration forces of over 100,000 times that due to the earth's gravity (g). These extreme forces are sufficient to centrifuge down even the smallest of the cell organelles.

Isolation of Cell Organelles in the Ultracentrifuge

The separation principle is simple: the bigger the cell organelle, the faster it sediments in the gravitation field of the ultracentrifuge. Nuclei, for example, can be spun down at only 800 g inside of 12 minutes. For the smaller mitochondria, 15,000 g and about 15 minutes are required. Thus, the cell organelles can be separated by size one after the other (Figure 21).

First, however, the cells must be broken up and the cell membranes destroyed, and here is where the problem lies. During destruction of the cell walls, the organelles should remain undamaged. Thus, many methods for preparing a cell brei are unsuitable for the isolation of organelles: if, for example, cells are swollen to bursting in a hypotonic salt solution, the membranes of the organelles suffer along with the outer membrane.

A proven and generally used method is the so-called Potter-Elvehjem homogenizer. This consists of a glass tube fitted with a movable pestle. While turning, the pestle is passed up and down in the tube: the cells are again and again forced between the glass wall and the pestle and are torn open by the shear forces developed. The much smaller cell organelles remain undamaged.

An even milder breaking method is possible with the so-called French press. First, the cells are subjected to a high nitrogen pressure in a pressure chamber. When this pressure is suddenly released, the resulting small gas bubbles tear open the cell membrane, again without any considerable influence on the organelles. (The same procedure used on a deep-sea diver causes "bends.")

Mild destruction of the cell membranes does not by itself guarantee undamaged cell organelles. The organelles must be isolated in as "natural" an environment as possible. Isotonic salt solutions and isotonic sucrose solutions are often used. In the meantime it has turned out that hypertonic sucrose solutions can be especially favorable for certain cell organelles. Traces of divalent cations such as calcium or magnesium can increase the stability of the organelles. Finally, a buffer must be used to ensure a neutral pH for the homogenate.

The Cell as a Chemical Factory

Even at the turn of the century, the cell was understood to be a "chemical factory." The production of glycogen and the excretion of urea in living cells are entirely analogous to the production of aniline dyes and sulfuric acid in industry. Apparently without effort the cell does things for which our chemical technology requires costly organization. Appearances are deceiving, however: in the cell, too, there is excruciating order: the widely differing metabolic paths are sharply separated from each other and develop next to each other.

The nucleus regulates production; it supplies the blueprints from which proteins are assembled on the ribosomes. The conveyor belts for protein production are in turn divided into stationary and mobile units: membrane-bound ribosomes (rough endoplasmic reticulum) and free ribosomes. The mitochondria specialize almost entirely in energy production.

Each of these organelles has been suspected of playing an especially important role in the development of a tumor cell.

- The prime suspect is the *nucleus,* which as the bearer of genetic material naturally stands at the center of all genetic cancer theories.
- This is followed by the *mitochondria,* which have their special interest in Warburg's cancer theory, as the seat of cell respiration.
- In the last few years, critical examination of the *cell membranes* has moved into the foreground. The membranes mediate contact between the single cells and thus their cohesion. But perhaps they are also important sensors of a cell, which receive regulatory impulses of the whole organism.
- Even the *lysosomes* don't get off scot free: Allison claims them to be the actual carcinogens, which are first activated by external carcinogens such as chemicals, radiations, or viruses.
- If we omit the *endoplasmic reticulum* (microsomes), this is done only for reasons of space. The reader could, however, look up recent work by H. C. Pitot and associates.
- Similarly, we will not discuss the role of the supernatant (the "S 3 fraction").

Let us now sketch out the possible roles of the single organelles in carcinogenesis, beginning with the nucleus.

The Nucleus and Carcinogenesis

If the nucleus is the steering organ of the cell, then the nucleus of a tumor cell would have to be responsible for the neoplastic properties of this cell. This simple conclusion found experimental support very early.

a) The altered chromosomal characteristics of many tumor cells are a direct indication of a change in the nucleus. But even invisible changes in the hereditary material of a somatic cell ("mutations") are, in the end, changes in the nucleus. In the chapter "Cancer and Inheritance" we will cover such changes more completely.

b) In the resting nucleus of a differentiated somatic cell (the so-called interphase nucleus), two morphologically different forms of the chromosomes can be identified. A few chromosome sections appear as *densely* packed "heterochromatin"; the remainder is present as *loosely* packed "euchromatin." These two forms of chromatin also differ in their biochemical activity: euchromatin synthesizes more RNA than heterochromatin, and actinomycin — a substance that ties up the synthesis of RNA at the DNA — is bound sixfold more by euchromatin than by heterochromatin.

In a somatic cell, the genetic information of the chromosomes is only partially decoded. In a liver cell, for example, all information must remain suppressed which would be peculiar to a nerve cell or a kidney cell. Thus, the chromosomes of a somatic cell contain active and inactive genes. Active genes and only active genes produce messenger RNA, thereby starting off production of specific enzymes that are finally responsible for the specific activities of a cell. The conclusion follows that euchromatin is associated with the active genes and heterochromatin with the inactive, repressed genes.

Euchromatin and heterochromatin can be distinguished not only under the microscope, but may also be separated on a preparative scale. Nuclei are sonicated and then centrifuged at different times and speeds. The heavy fraction, obtained after short, low-speed centrifugation (1,000 g, 10 minutes) consists primarily of heterochromatin. The light fraction (78,000 g, 60 minutes) contains predominantly euchromatin.

During diethylnitrosamine carcinogenesis, the proportion of heterochromatin in a liver cell increases, and after 40 days the increase amounts to about 20 percent (Harbers). The "active" euchromatin decreased correspondingly. In contrast, the total DNA content of the cell remains constant. This means that the available genetic information is limited during tumor development. The number of active genes decreases. Early findings on the depletion of organ specific enzymes in tumors fit into this picture, for the loss of euchromatin means a loss of organ-specific synthetic capabilities.

From this viewpoint, carcinogenesis is seen to be a "heterochromatization" (Sandritter): the genetic program of a cell is obviously sent oft in a new direction. At this point, let us put off further discussion until we can discuss the most important tumor theories together.

c) Besides the DNA, the most important component of the chromosomes may be the so-called *histones*. These are proteins with high levels of lysine and arginine. The high proportion of these basic amino acids permits a close "salt-like" bond between acidic DNA and basic histones.

Because of this, it was long believed that it could be just these histones which cover certain DNA regions and thus "inactivate." To be sure, difficulties appeared when the histones were more carefully analyzed and it was discovered that there are only about 10 different types of histones (which can be separated by acrylamide electrophoresis). How are these few histones supposed to be capable of specifically blocking thousands of different pieces of genetic information on a DNA fiber?

Today molecular biologists are inclined to believe that specific RNA, together with specific repressor proteins, decide where and when DNA is blocked. The histones then take over a more permanent blocking role.

Nonetheless, a few authors have discovered differences between histones of normal cells and tumor cells. Busch reported a histone fraction (RP2-L) which he found only in Walker carcinoma cells, but not in normal cells. Attempts to demonstrate this unusual histone in other tumor cells were without success, however.

The role of the nucleus for a tumor cell thus remains unclear to a great extent. There is no lack of hints, but proof is lacking; still, we seem to be on the right track. According to all experience, the neoplastic properties of a tumor cell are hereditary, and the nucleus is primarily responsible for the transmission of hereditary properties.

Lysosomes

De Duve has called the lysosomes "suicide packages." These cell particles are barely smaller than small mitochondria and were thus discovered relatively late. They contain a "balled-up charge" of hydrolytic enzymes, which can cleave proteins and nucleic acids, among other things. Normally these self-destructive instruments are safely shut up in the lysosomes. If the cell is damaged, however, they can be set free and effectively take part in elimination of the cell debris. Thus, lysosomes seem to play an important role in inflammatory reactions. Observations by Allison brought the lysosomes into the purview of cancer research.

Carcinogenic Hydrocarbons are Taken up by Lysosomes

Allison pursued the uptake of polycyclic hydrocarbons into living cells. For this he used tissue culture cells — in order to exclude indirect effects — and made use of polynuclear hydrocarbons, because they can be easily detected with a fluorescence microscope. This direct microscopic method avoids possible exchange of carcinogenic substances between cell organelles during homogenization and fractionation of the cells.

Under the fluorescence microscope, the cell nuclei remained dark, but the cytoplasm lit up in ultraviolet light. Graffi had supposed that mitochondria were involved, but Allison could show that it is the lysosomes which fluoresce; fluorescence and the localization of lysosomal (hydrolytic) enzymes are in agreement. Allison believed that the carcinogens liberate lysosomal DNases, which in turn attack nuclear DNA.

Lysosomal DNases as Carcinogens

Lysosomes do in fact contain a DNase which can cleave double-stranded DNA, breaking both strands. It is even possible in a test tube to break down isolated chromosomes with this enzyme. Chromosome breaks can be induced in vivo, too, if the lysosomes are damaged, which can be done selectively with a surprisingly simple technique.

If living cells are treated with Neutral Red, only the lysosomes are stained. If these cells with the "red lysosomes" are irradiated with green light (which is absorbed by the red particles), the lysosomes can then be selectively set off (photosensitization).

If Allison's ideas are right, then a normally harmless dye, combined with light of appropriate wavelength, ought to be *carcinogenic*. On photosensitization of hamster kidney cells in tissue culture, Allison occasionally observed transformed cells. "Our investigations suggest quite strongly that lysosomal damage *can* produce malignant transformation in cells, or facilitate transformation occurring spontaneously." It should not be surprising that transformation in vitro using photosensitization has not shown any convincing successes. Transformation in a test tube is in general problematic. Leaving transformation by oncogenic viruses out of the picture, "artificial" production of tumor cells in vitro is difficultly attainable, and even proven carcinogens easily fail us in such efforts.

It really ought to be easier to stain the skin of a mouse red and then irradiate it. For such a red mouse, green light ought to be a carcinogenic stimulus. This experiment has not yet been done, but there is a very similar example from human medicine: porphyria. In this case, too, the skin of the patients is oversensitive to normal light to a high degree. Misformed pigments (porphyrins) have sensitized the cells. From the base of severe skin damage arise malignant tumors. (As early as the 1930's, Büngeler was able to show that this disease can be imitated in animals: if mice are subjected to intensive exposure to sunlight, they develop skin tumors more frequently if they are also treated with eosin or hematoporphyrin.)

Unfortunately, all findings do not fit into a thought system without any gaps. The worst hole is the finding that noncarcinogenic substances (anthracene, for example) are also taken up by lysosomes. Nonetheless, the number of fingers pointing at the lysosomes is increasing, and consequently we cannot exclude the possibility that these particles play a greater role in carcinogenesis than was previously assumed.

Cell Membranes, Cell Sociology, and Carcinogenesis

It all began with a chance observation: it struck Coman that tumor cells can be separated from each other more easily than can normal cells. He had made this observation as he was trying to separate epidermal cells with a micromanipulator. It had turned out that tumor cells form a looser cell organization than normal cells; they are less "attached"; their social behavior appears to be fundamentally disturbed.

Therefore, we are going to pursue a bit of practical cell sociology and more closely examine contacts between single cells. The cell membranes are responsible for these contacts, and thus our report on cell sociology necessarily becomes a report also on the surface properties of tumor cells.

Cell Sociology in Tissue Culture

Cells in a culture bottle or a petri dish migrate actively across the glass bottom. If such a migrating cell meets another cell, contact usually takes place. This contact then stops further isolated movement of the cell.

But not only the motion of the cell is blocked. Radical alterations in metabolism can take place, with the end result that DNA synthesis is shut off and further cell division becomes impossible.

This inhibition of cell division by cell contact is often called "contact inhibition." This contact inhibition offers an effective guard against overpopulation in tissue culture: if the cells grow to a continuous "turf" of cells, in which each cell is surrounded by other cells, then there is no more division.

Tumor cells behave otherwise: they migrate over their neighbor cells — entirely as if they were simply glass — and do not stop dividing when they have reached confluence (grown together). Obviously, tumor cells are blind to each other, and the preventive measure against overpopulation has failed.

The behavior in the animal corresponds to this behavior in the bottle: tumor cells with disturbed contact inhibition in vitro show malignant, invasive growth in vivo; the unsocial behavior in the animal corresponds to the unsocial behavior in culture.

Membrane Changes in Tumor Cells

The disturbed social behavior of tumor cells is mirrored in altered cell membranes. A simple method for getting a first look at the properties of these membranes is the electrophoresis of whole cells. The cells under investigation are suspended in a suitable medium in a transparent chamber. Using a microscope, one then observes the movement of these cells under the influence of an electrical field. With a stopwatch the rate of migration of the cells is measured. This rate is primarily dependent on the charge density of the cell surface.

With this method cell suspensions from solid tumors (kidney carcinomas, hepatomas) were investigated and compared with cells from the normal parent tissue. It turned out that the tumor cells were more negatively charged than the corresponding normal cells. Figure 22 gives an example of such a Pherogram (Ambrose): shown is the percentage of cells in the total population with their respectively indicated mobilities.

Polyoma-transformed cells also differ from nontransformed fibroblasts by an elevated "negative mobility." Ruthenstroth-Bayer obtained similar results in an investigation of leukemia cells: granulocytes or lymphocytes were respectively replaced, according to the type of leukemia, by more rapidly migrating cells.

Malignancy of a tumor cell and its migration rate in an electrical field seem to be connected: Ambrose analyzed cells from a tumor series in which a solid tumor, a metastasizing tumor, and also an ascites tumor were represented (all tumors derived from the same original tumor). In this series the binding forces between the individual cells decrease, until they are especially small in the ascites cells, which grow isolated from each other. The excess negative charge, however, increased in the same order (Figure 22).

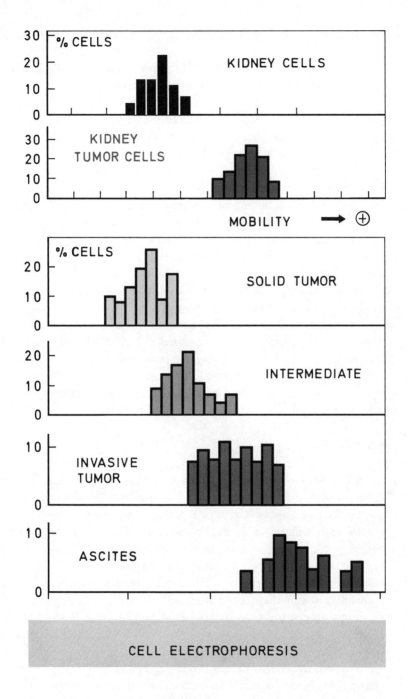

Figure 22

Neuraminic Acid and Phospholipids "Negativize" Cell Membranes

Indirect methods permitted inferences as to the substances which cause the excessive negative charges of the tumor cells.

1. If cells are treated with the enzyme neuraminidase, neuraminic acid is cleaved off without destruction of the cell membranes. Such neuraminidase-treated cells are less mobile in an electrical field and can lose as much as 90 percent of their excess negative charge.

2. Phospholipids of the cell membranes bind calcium ions. Cell membranes covered up with calcium ions are similarly less negatively charged, and the cells migrate correspondingly slower. (The tentative identification of phospholipids as bearers of negative charge was obtained using model compounds and a more exact analysis of the pH dependency of both cell mobility and the charge on synthetic phospholipids.)

3. Recently nucleic acids have also been suspected of contributing to the negative charge on cell membranes.

In certain leukemia cells almost the entire charge excess can be removed with neuraminidase. For Ehrlich ascites cells obviously other anions are important. The greater mobility of polyoma-transformed cells as against nontransformed cells again might rest almost exclusively on neuraminic acid: after neuraminidase treatment, the mobility is reduced to the value of normal fibroblasts.

Binding Forces between Cells

"A society of hedgehogs," Schopenhauer once wrote, "crowded close together one cold winter day, to protect themselves from freezing by their neighbors' warmth. But they soon felt their mutual sticking of each other, which drove them apart again. Now when the necessity for warmth again brought them together, this second evil repeated itself, so that they were thrown from one suffering to the other, until they eventually worked out a reasonable separation from each other which they could best put up with." Binding forces and repulsion forces together determine the distance of hedgehog from hedgehog. Binding and repulsion must also be balanced out between single cells.

Charges of the same sign on the cell surfaces are primarily responsible for *repulsion*. The excess negative charges on the one partner repel the negative charges of the other (Coulomb's law).

Binding forces are composed of several components: besides complementary surface structures, calcium ions are primarily decisive. These divalent ions connect the single cells into giant complexes. The calcium can be dissolved out from between the cells with compounds like ethylenediamine tetraacetic acid (EDTA). EDTA has a stronger affinity for calcium ions than do the negative structures of the cell surfaces, and thus a calcium complex ("chelate") of EDTA is formed. Embryos of amphibians can, as an example, be broken up into single cells by such an EDTA treatment. The separation of such embryonic cells is reversible; after addition of calcium, the cells reaggregate and even continue their interrupted embryonic development.

Normally, however, cells are not simply connected with calcium bridges. Normal adult cells excrete substances into the intercellular spaces which assist the cells to stick to each other. Agglutinated cells can naturally no longer be separated by chelating agents. Stronger measures are necessary, which can dissolve the protein-containing mediator substances. Normally one uses trypsin. Thus, with 0.4 percent trypsin solution at 37 °C, small pieces of tissue can be separated into single cells. This trypsinization has become today one of the most important standard methods in tissue culture laboratories. It requires a very delicate touch, for if the pieces of tissue are digested too long, the cells are then more or less severely damaged.

All in all, the following picture results: "In the formation of intercellular adhesions, the Coulomb repulsive forces appear to be overcome in local regions by links involving calcium ions. Subsequently, the contacts become stabilized by protein secretion from within the cells" (Ambrose).

Cell Contacts are Specific

Cells are choosy. Strong bonds do not form between all cells: they must suit each other. The first clear indications of cell-specific binding derived from experiments with sponges. Sponges can be dissociated into single cells and then later reaggregated. Now, sponges of different strains were dissociated into single cells and these cells mixed together. Upon reaggregation the cells again separated: only cells of the same strain assembled into cell complexes; mixed sponges were not formed.

Even mammalian cells avoid contact with foreign cells; if rat tissue is placed in a culture of mouse organs, the rat tissue largely isolates itself from the mouse tissue.

Finally, Moscona was able to prove that even cells of individual organs can recognize each other. From a mixture of kidney cells and liver cells, the liver and kidney cells sorted themselves out and formed separate aggregates, whose fine structures even resembled the original intact organs. (See Figure 23.)

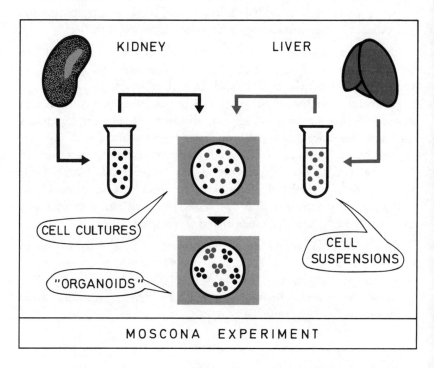

Figure 23

Normal Cells can Regulate Tumor Cells

Ascites tumor cells are born loners: they reproduce in peritoneal fluid as if they were one-celled organisms. Their excess negative charge offers a simple explanation: the electrostatic repulsion forces predominate over possibly present tendencies toward aggregation.

Even these loners, however, can be outwitted: on shaking of ascites fluid — according to Moscona — for an extended period (33 days) compact aggregates form with mesenchymal and epithelial components (Schleich). The histology of such tumor organoids can under certain conditions even give away the origin of unknown ascites tumor cells.

The extended shaking technique also gave surprising results with HeLa cells: these cells grow in tissue culture as a monolayer. On shaking with mesenchymal cells, however, here multicellular aggregates were formed, regardless of whether these mesenchymal cells came from chickens, rats, or even from man. Interactions between normal and neoplastic cells thus certainly play a large role in the behavior of tumor cells.

Stoker studied these interactions in another example: he added polyoma-transformed fibroblasts to a culture of normal contact-inhibited fibroblasts. While polyoma-transformed cells show all the typical signs of neoplastic growth ("criss-cross and piling up") among themselves, the transformed cells in the mixed culture arranged them-

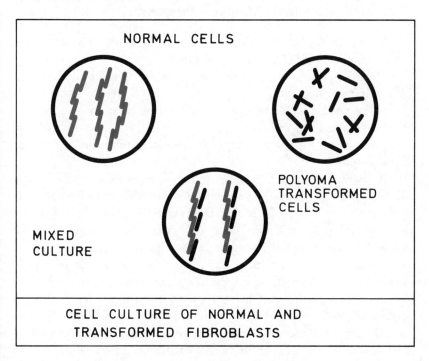

Figure 24

selves parallel to the non-transformed cells (Figure 24). Their growth rate is simultaneously blocked.

From this Stoker concludes that normal cells can send out and receive contact signals, which then determine association and growth rate of the cells. Tumor cells, on the other hand, can no longer send signals, but they can still receive them. Thus, tumor cells grow uncontrolled among themselves; tumor cells which still have contacts with normal cells can, in contrast, still be "controlled."

Sending and receiving does not have to mean that signals are actually sent out, possibly as signal substances produced by the cells and also taken up by them. Direct, specifically complementary surface contacts are more plausible, and with such structures, too, it is possible to construct models for "sender and receiver."

These findings illustrate again that a single tumor cell is really not a tumor cell. Only when enough neoplastic cells have collected in a tumor cell nest, can they escape from the regulation of the parent tissue ("critical mass" of tumor cell colonies).

Carcinogenesis From the Membrane Perspective

To conclude, let us once more sketch the path to a tumor cell from the viewpoint of the cell membranes:

a) development of a changed cell membrane, which hinders close cell contact, and

b) aggregation of many contact-disturbed cells, which facilitates release from cell organization.

The excessive negative charge of tumor cells offers an explanation for both phases.

A change in the cell membrane alone, however — and even the disturbed social behavior — cannot be responsible for carcinogenesis, for normal cells too can escape from a cell organization. The best known example is the blood-forming system. In this tissue cells are formed which loosen their connections with their neighbors, finally leave the tissue organization, and float out into the circulation as single cells. In this manner granulocytes, lymphocytes, and other blood cells are supplied. Obviously, changes quite similar to those in carcinogenesis are involved in the maturation of these cells.

Changed cell membranes and altered social behavior can therefore not be the only cause for development of a tumor cell. It is most assuredly however a significant necessity for autonomous growth.

A Small Natural Philosophy of Cell Membranes

It is only through membranes that a cell obtains its individuality. The "coacervates" which, according to Oparin, swam around in the primeval mud were therefore still not cells. There could only be cells after cell membranes were "invented." These membranes are thus at the beginning of the cell story.

In the course of evolution they have undergone great changes. They have long since outgrown their first assignment of defining cells from each other. Today cell membranes are more than inert coverings for a droplet of protoplasm. They decide on uptake and release of substances important to the cell. They help the cell to actively convey to its interior substances which it requires, and to enrich its supply. Membranes guarantee a constant "milieu interieur" to such a cell. The high potassium ion concentrations of a mammalian cell in a low potassium environment are a well-known example of this "milieu cellulaire."

A tumor cell becomes increasingly foreign to its neighbors; tumor cells can no longer recognize each other in their altered cell membranes. Yet the changed membranes do not signify changed surface properties only. Membrane alterations can interfere far into the inner structures of a cell. A higher cell can be understood as a complicated system of layers and network. Robertson once presented a clear picture of the developmental series from a simple to a highly differentiated cell (Figure 25). Changes in this system consequently do not affect simply the outer membrane layers.

Thus, for a single cell, cell membranes occupy a key position. This great significance gave rise to the suspicion that cell membranes can reproduce themselves. The sentence *"Omnis cellula e cellula"* would accordingly be read not only as *Omne DNA e DNA,* but also as *Omnis Membrana e Membrana.*

The replication of cell membranes under their own management would naturally not mean that the membranes also construct their own building blocks. The recent discovery of microsomal DNA makes the question again appear an open one, to be sure, but autonomous replication signifies only that membranes are capable of putting together the raw materials supplied by the cell, according to their own requirements. The membrane structure could establish simple association rules (white binds black, black binds white). This simple model also makes it possible to understand how a single disturbance,

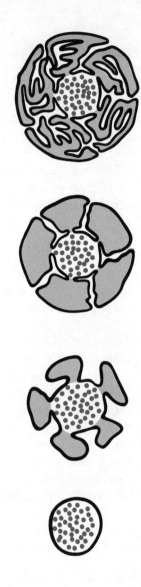

EVOLUTION OF MEMBRANES

Figure 25

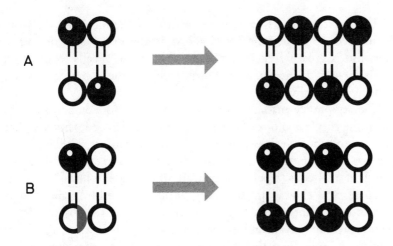

MODEL OF MEMBRANE REPLICATION

Figure 26

possibly by a carcinogen, can lead to a permanently modified membrane structure (Figure 26).

Indications of such "membrane mutants" have been found in Paramecia (Sonneborn), but as yet there has been no similar finding in mammalian cells.

The concept of self-replicating membranes has fascinating consequences: the construction of a tumor cell would be possible without having to bother the nucleus. A "neoplastic alteration" of the cell membranes would also be "inherited" by the daughter cells without the necessity of a DNA change.

Is there Really a "Contact Inhibition"? Growth Factors vs. Contact Inhibition

Until now we have assumed that contact inhibition really does derive primarily from contact between cells: cells grow until contact on all sides keeps them from growing further.

In the organism, cell divisions in a tissue appear to be held under control by inhibitors produced in the tissue ("chalones"). If we transfer this concept to cell cultures, it would mean that one would have to look for inhibitors given off by resting cells and capable of specifically blocking cell division.

This search appears to be unsuccessful for the moment. Cells can be cultured on membrane filters. Now if the upper side of such a filter disc is grown full, it is still possible for new cells to grow on the underside. Hence, the confluent cells on the top side are not releasing any inhibitors.

The regulatory mechanism of intact tissue thus seems to play no role in the regulation of cell division in culture. This does not say that contact inhibition derives primarily from cell contact. Holley found a trivial solution to the problem when he investigated closely the growth of 3T3-cells (a permanent strain of mouse fibroblasts).

These cells exhibit an especially beautiful case of "contact inhibition": under normal culture conditions these cells grow quickly to a confluent monolayer, and as soon as this stage is reached, they stop growing. At this point they reach a cell density of about one million cells per petri dish (6 cm diameter).

It was noticed early, however — and not only for 3T3 cells — that, upon addition of fresh medium with fresh calf serum, a new wave of mitosis is induced even in a confluent culture. From this one was forced to conclude that growth factors in the calf serum could override contact inhibition.

Holley then found that the characteristic cell density of a "contact inhibited" culture is only the chance result of nutrient concentration. 3T3 cells grow to varying final concentrations depending on the proportion of serum in the medium (Figure 27).

At 6×10^6 cells/dish, the cultures became confluent independently of the serum concentration. This event is not noticeable in the growth curves.

Consequently, one or more growth factors in the calf serum appear to be primarily decisive for the final cell count of a 3T3 culture. When this factor is used up by the cells, growth stops.

It follows then that 3T3 cells do not grow in an "exhausted" medium (Figure 27): if one takes the medium from a stationary culture and adds it to other 3T3 cells, no cell division follows. Only the addition of fresh calf serum permits new division.

Tumor cells behave entirely otherwise: SV-40-transformed 3T3 cells grow even in "exhausted" media. Hence, the growth factor requirement of these cells has been considerably reduced. Quite similar observations have been made on cultures of chicken fibroblasts (Temin): normal fibroblasts require a serum factor, but fibroblasts

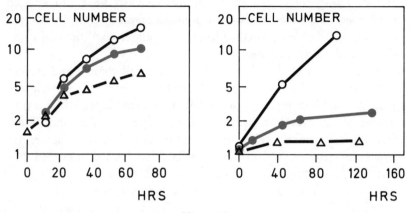

Figure 27

transformed by Rous sarcoma virus get along with much less serum factor.

Accordingly, a decisive difference between a normal cell and a tumor cell in tissue culture is found in differing requirements for growth factor. Whether cell contact is involved is secondary.

But it is still too early to decide whether we must replace "contact inhibition" by "growth factors" in our thinking. Even taken together, growth factors and membrane control do not seem to be the whole story.

Inhibitors Guarantee "Contact Inhibition"

For the moment, let us continue to focus our attention on 3T3 cells, which show contact inhibition especially well. What happens if we grow these cells in a culture in which the medium is constantly replenished (perfusion culture)?

If growth factors alone determine the maximum attainable cell density, then the 3T3 cells ought to continue to grow under such luxury conditions, piling up and eventually forming multilayered cultures. This is exactly what does not happen. Castor made motion pictures of 3T3 perfusion cultures and saw that only monolayers are formed. Using time-lapse photography, he saw what Holley had already seen, that these cells could squeeze together after initial contact, but still shut off growth. Hence, even under conditions of overflowing, cell count is limited.

What is it, then, that limits cell growth if cell contact and growth factors are not the whole story? The following is a suggestive hypothesis: contact between cells in a sufficiently dense layer initiates production of an inhibitor which stops cell division. Yeh and Fisher presented experiments which support the idea that such factors are actually present in "old media" (media from contact-inhibited cultures). By replacing the medium in a confluent culture with fresh medium, an additional mitosis could be induced in about 6 percent of the cells. Surprisingly, it was also possible to initiate these "forbidden" cell divisions with the following treatment: the "old medium" was first replaced by physiological saline, which in turn was replaced by the original old medium.

This apparently remarkable finding can be understood if one assumes an inhibitor: the saline dilutes out an inhibitor and the cells prepare themselves for a new round of division. The first steps for new DNA synthesis and subsequent mitosis are set in motion (primarily involving RNA, according to Yeh and Fisher), but in saline the cells cannot get very far because of the lack of nutrients. These are supplied by the old medium which replaces the saline. Of course, the inhibitor is still present, but since the process leading to division had already been initiated, the inhibitor was without effect on the immediate mitosis. (The inhibiting principle is of low molecular weight and is lost upon dialysis of old medium.)

These findings contradict those of the Millipore experiment described above, which showed that confluent cells do not release inhibitors of growing cells. Yet this contradiction is superficial: Yeh and Fisher's inhibitor need not be required to inhibit growing cells. Its job is to maintain contact inhibition, so that it should not be surprising that it cannot inhibit cells which are not in contact. (We should point out that some cells, such as the human fibroblasts WI-38 investigated by Garcia-Giratt, obviously do produce substances which also inhibit growing cells.)

Consideration of these investigations leads us directly to the chalone concept (see page 77). Chalones are also inhibitors, which affect cells in the contacts of a tissue (ignoring the questionable leukemia chalone). Chalone concentration is dependent on the mass of tissue, as noted previously, and a similar mechanism is possibly operative in tissue culture: when the cell count has reached a certain limiting density, the inhibitor concentration is sufficient to brake the entire population.

Growth regulation in tissue culture, as artificial as it might seem on first glance, therefore has obvious similarities to growth regulation in the intact organ in vivo. But this was really to be expected, for the behavior of cells in tissue culture permits inferences concerning the behavior of these cells in the animal: tumor cells that do not fit into a prescribed order in vivo also are not subject to the rules of "contact inhibition" in cell cultures.

Let us now try to summarize once more those factors that determine maximal population density of a tissue culture, even if the story may not be complete:

a) growth factors alone are out of the question,
b) inhibitors alone do not suffice, and even
c) cell contact by itself is obviously insufficient.

Still it is certain that this contact and the cell membranes play an important role in the decision as to whether cells are mutually inhibitory or not. Certainly there is more than a superficial distinction between the membranes of tumor cells and normal cells, more than the simple differences which have already been catalogued (Ca binding, neuraminic acid content, etc.). Recently, however, there was success in finding a difference between the membranes of tumor cells and normal cells that may be directly related to growth properties. Put simply, a reason was found why tumor cells grow without contact inhibition, while normal cells fit into the "culture's order."

Membranes Regulate Cell Growth

By 1963 it had already been discovered that wheat germ contains certain substances which can cause "clumping" of tumor cells (Aub). These *agglutinins* operate similarly to antibodies: they have (at least) two binding sites and can therefore react with (at least) two cells and cause agglutination (clumping) (Figure 28). By 1963, Aub had already found that primarily tumor cells can be agglutinated and that hardly any normal cells are.

In succeeding years, workers occupied themselves primarily with an agglutinating protein from jack beans which Sumner had already

NORMAL CELLS + CON A

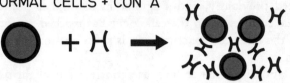 NO AGGLU-
TINATION

TUMOR CELLS + CON A

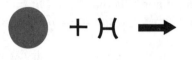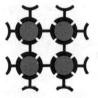 AGGLU-
TINATION

TUMOR CELLS + "CON A"/2

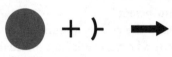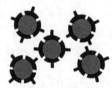 NO AGGLU-
TINATION

NORMAL CELLS IN CULTURE

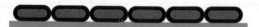

TUMOR CELLS IN CULTURE

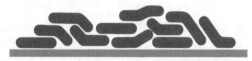

TUMOR CELLS + CON A/2 IN CULTURE

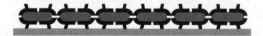

Figure 28

112

crystallized in the 1930's, Concanavalin A (Con A). Con A is similarly specific for tumor cells. However, not only tumor cells can be agglutinated: if normal 3T3 cells are treated with a dilute solution of the protein-cleaving enzyme trypsin, they then bind Con A just as do transformed 3T3 cells. Obviously, the trypsinization had laid bare in normal cells the same binding sites that are always exposed in tumor cells. In other words, in normal cells there are binding sites covered that are uncovered in tumor cells.

This led to a simple question: what happens if these binding sites are covered in tumor cells; do the cells again become "normal"? Some trickery was required to answer this question, since Con A had to be able to cover the binding sites without agglutinating the cells. Hence, a "one-armed," monovalent Con A was required, which could react with only one cell. Such could easily be prepared, however: trypsin cleaves Con A into fragments that can still react with tumor cells, but which can no longer agglutinate them (Burger).

Now, if tumor cells are treated with monovalent Con A, they survive this procedure very well. They continue to divide in cell culture, but (here was the surprise) only until a confluent cell layer is attained, at which point they stop growing. In other words, Con A had converted them to normal cells, again subject to contact inhibition. They had become wolves in sheep's clothing.

Wolves they remained, nonetheless: the binding of monovalent Con A is reversible. Excess methylglucose, for example, competes for the Con A and in this way again detaches it from the cell membrane. Now the tumor cells make their appearance again, growing regardless of contacts in the cell culture, as they did before the Con A episode.

This does not finish the Con A story, however. If it is correct that the binding sites for Con A are important for growth behavior, then the trypsin-treated, Con A-binding 3T3 cells that we have just referred to must also be "tumor" cells. And, in fact, it was possible to release contact-inhibited cells from contact inhibition by trypsinization, to induce a new round of DNA synthesis with subsequent cell division. Trypsin can *remove* normal *growth properties* only on a short-term basis, however. Once each cell has divided again, cell divisions are shut off. They also fail to bind Con A any more: they were only "interim" tumor cells.

We can conclude this chapter by asking what these sites mean. Chemically, at least, the answer appears to be simple: they are probably glycoproteins with glucose as a component of the specific binding group, since Burger found that α-methylglucose competes with the cells to bind Con A, thus releasing the cells from Con A inhibition.

What function do these membrane structures have? Consider once more the concept which says that normal cells in tissue culture can both produce and respond to growth-regulating impulses. One might

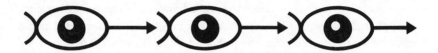

conclude that virus-transformed cells (SV40-3T3) are unable to exchange signals and thus grow without contact inhibition. This sup-

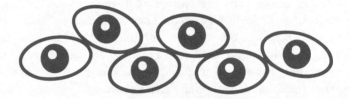

position is false, for the behavior of mixed cultures of normal cells and tumor cells (page 102) showed that tumor cells are entirely capable of receiving regulatory signals from normal cells. Thus, they have forgotten how to send, but not how to receive.

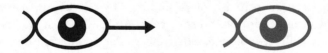

Concanavalin A makes the "sending" again possible, a phenomenon that is explained with difficulty by postulating simple covering of otherwise open binding sites. The whole sender-receiver concept could be false, of course. But possibly Con A simply indirectly covers the negative surface charges which make cell contact difficult and which force tumor cells to grow without contact inhibition.

Summary

Besides the nucleus and the lysosomes, the cell membranes appear to be especially important organelles in carcinogenesis. All three together offer a complete theory for the development of a tumor cell:

1. Lysosomal enzymes, especially lysosomal DNase, alter the DNA in the nucleus.

2. The altered DNA produces "more acid" membrane building blocks than normal DNA. The negative cell membrane changes the social properties of a cell.

Up to this point we have ignored a particularly important cell organelle, the mitochondrion. But it is exactly the mitochondria — as claimed by Warburg's theory of cancer — that alone are in a position to permit development of a tumor cell. We must therefore direct our close attention to this organelle.

THE MITOCHONDRIA AND WARBURG'S CANCER THEORY

The mitochondria — the power plants of a cell — stand at the center of one of the oldest biochemical tumor theories; this theory sees the actual requirement for malignant growth in the damage to cell respiration and in "aerobic glycolysis." In 1923, Otto Warburg discovered glycolysis by tumors; in 1955 he collected observations and hypotheses into a suggestive mental structure.

Energy Production in the Respiratory Chain

The so-called respiratory chain is localized in the mitochondria. It consists of several enzymes working in succession which "burn" with oxygen the hydrogen stemming from nutrients. For our purposes it is sufficient now to imagine this respiratory chain as a black box into which one feeds O_2 and H_2 (as the reduced coenzyme NADH) and which supplies remarkable amounts of energy (ATP) along with water.

Glycolysis

In the breakdown of glucose to pyruvic acid, ATP is produced directly, i. e., without intervention of the respiratory chain. (Consult a biochemistry text for exact details.) Compared to the high production caused by oxidative phosphorylation in the respiratory chain, this ATP production is minor, but this minor ATP output guarantees energy production even without oxygen.

There are problems, however: for every glucose molecule that is eventually broken down to pyruvic acid, two molecules of NAD must take on hydrogen, thus being reduced to NADH. The supply of NAD in the cell is limited, however, and thus the breakdown of glucose would eventually have to come to a halt. Only when the NADH formed can be recycled can glucose catabolism continue.

This retrieval of NAD is taken care of by lactate dehydrogenase, an enzyme which converts pyruvic acid to lactic acid:

$$\underset{O}{\underset{\|}{CH_3CCOOH}} \quad \underset{\overset{\longleftarrow}{NAD}}{\overset{NADH}{}} \quad \underset{OH}{\underset{|}{CH_3CHCOOH}}$$

One molecule of NAD is freed with each molecule of lactic acid, permitting throughput of another half a molecule of glucose. The path from glucose to lactic acid is called lactate glycolysis; by this method as much glucose as required can be converted to "energy" without oxygen.

Glycolysis is a poor substitute for respiration however: only 52 kcal/mole of glucose are produced (2 moles ATP). With respiration 686 kcal/mole of glucose can be obtained (38 moles ATP).

Warburg's Manometric Methods for Measurement of Respiration and Glycolysis

Oxygen is consumed during respiration: if one then connects a culture vessel containing cells (cell suspension, tissue slices) to a manometer, one can directly read oxygen consumption. Warburg defined a respiratory coefficient Q_{O_2} as the number of cubic millimeters of oxygen consumed by 1 mg of tissue (dry weight) at oxygen saturation and $38°$ C in 1 hour.

The manometric method was also applied to the measurement of lactic acid by Warburg. Each mole of lactic acid releases a mole of

CO_2 from a bicarbonate buffer, and this can be measured mano-metrically. Here, too, a quotient can be defined ($Q_M^{N_2}$ or $Q_M^{O_2}$), which tells how many cubic millimeters of CO_2 are released by a milligram of tissue in 1 hour. The superscript N_2 or O_2 indicates whether the measurement was done under nitrogen (anaerobic) or oxygen (aerobic).

Cancer Cells Glycolyze

The high glycolysis of ascites cells was discovered in Berlin-Dahlem (1952) in Warburg's laboratory, and has since then been repeatedly confirmed. But even in 1923 Warburg had measured oxygen consumption and lactic acid production on slices from solid tumors and found that they consumed less oxygen and produced more lactic acid than normal tissue.

The respiration of cancer cells is obviously damaged. Does this mean that respiratory damage leads to tumor development?

Carcinogens Damage Respiration

.An injury to respiration that leads to tumor development must fulfill two rigorous criteria:

1. It must lead to an irreversible injury, for the originally damaged respiration remains damaged throughout succeeding cell divisions.

2. The injury must not kill the cell. It is consequently not to be expected that all respiratory poisons are also carcinogens.

The equality respiratory poison = carcinogen should be capable of reversal: all carcinogens ought to injure respiration. *Nitrosamines* fit into this picture, and the classical carcinogenic *hydrocarbons* are no exception. Respiration is also destroyed by *X-ray* irradiation: "Evidently carcinogenesis by X-rays is nothing but the destruction of respiration by eliminating respiring mitochondria" (Warburg, as are the following quotations).

Simple respiratory damage does not yet cause cancer: "If a destruction of respiration is supposed to cause cancer, this destruction, as already mentioned must be irreversible." Warburg proposed an elegant solution for this problem: it is only necessary to assume that mitochondria are independent microorganisms, which reproduce independently of the nucleus. Then a mitochondrion can arise only from a mitochondrion. The result is that a cell in which the mitochondria are "shot down" cannot form any new mitochondria. Naturally, the same holds true for the daughter cells.

Omne Granum e Grano

The autoreplication of the "respiratory grana" had long since been postulated. From purely morphological considerations — the mitochondria are isolated, complex structured particles — it had been concluded that mitochondria really ought to be considered symbionts.

Impressive indications of this symbiotic status have been produced very recently. The mitochondria contain their own DNA and are thus in a position to realize their own blueprints (in RNA).

Path to the Tumor Cell: Selection of Cells Capable of Glycolysis

"Even if the respiration of somatic cells has become irreversibly damaged, there has been no appearance of cancer cells, for in order for cancer cells to arise, we require not only irreversible injury to respiration, but also a rise in glycolysis, in particular, an increase sufficient to make up energetically for the lost respiration. But how does this rise in glycolysis come about?"

If DAB or diethylnitrosamine is fed to rats, after a long latent period the glycolysis of the liver increases to the value characteristic for tumors.

The driving force for this rise in glycolysis is the energy deficiency which results from destruction of respiration and compels the cells to replace somehow the irretrievably lost respiration energy. They do this (as a population) by a selection process which makes use of the glycolysis of the normal somatic cells. The more weakly glycolyzing cells perish, the more strongly glycolyzing cells survive, and this selection process continues until the respiration loss has been energetically compensated for by the rise in glycolysis. Only then has a cancer cell arisen from a normal cell. Furthermore, we understand why the rise in glycolysis takes so long, and why it is only possible with the aid of many cell divisions.

Glycolytic Energy is "Inferior"

"Why, and this is our last question, do somatic cells become de-differentiated when their respiratory energy is replaced by glycolytic energy?" Glycolysis as well as respiration supplies ATP in the end, and ATP really ought to be ATP.

Warburg shores up his thesis of the inferior energy of glycolysis with two arguments, historical and morphological.

> Geology teaches us that there were life forms on earth before there was oxygen in the atmosphere. These organisms living without oxygen were glycolyzing, little differentiated single celled organisms. Only when free oxygen entered the atmosphere — about 800 million years ago — did the higher development of life enter the picture, almost suddenly, and the plant and animal kingdoms arose. The "evolution creatrice" is thus the work of oxygen, or to put it more exactly: the work of oxygen respiration.
>
> The reverse pathway of dedifferentiation of highly developed somatic cells takes place today most prominently in cancer induction.

Carcinogenesis appears to be a "relapse" into primitive growth customs.

In addition to this historical analogy, Warburg clarifies the "inferiority of glycolytic energy" with the following train of throught: the respiratory chain is localized in the mitochondria, the glycolytic enzymes in the cytoplasm. The ATP formed by respiration is thus synthesized in a structured organelle and consequently is imbued with more "structure" than ATP synthesized via glycolysis. "It is as if one were to illuminate two photographic plates with the same amount of light, with diffuse light in one case and with ordered light in the other. In the one case there results a diffuse blackening, in the other a picture." One is reminded of the philosophical dictum that order can arise only out of order.

Oxygen Deficiency in Tumor Tissue

Under oxygen deficiency cancer cells have a considerable advantage over normal cells: their glycolysis helps them to survive while normal cells must die without oxygen.

Tumor cells cannot grow without any oxygen, to be sure, but in a tumor the partial pressure of oxygen is usually lower than that necessary for normal cells. The low level of oxygen in a tumor can be demonstrated with a simple experiment: if tetanus spores are injected into mice, the mice remain healthy. The anaerobic tetanus spores can germinate only under oxygen deficiency, and the oxygen pressure is not low enough in any tissue of the mouse to make this possible. If the anaerobic tetanus spores are injected into tumor-bearing mice, however, the animals sicken, for now the spores find in the tumor a milieu with a low oxygen level. This experiment proves that tumor cells not only *can* grow anaerobically, but that they actually *do* grow anaerobically in tumors (Malmgren).

This spore-tumor effect can be utilized *therapeutically* (Moese): if one treats a tumor host with appropriate anaerobic spores, the growing bacteria settle in the tumors and there selectively destroy the tumor tissue. The tumors soften and finally break up.

Tumor Development in Two Phases

Warburg summarizes his respiration theory of cancer in apodictic sentences:

Cancer cells arise from normal somatic cells in two phases. The *first* phase is the irreversible damage of respiration. As there are many peripheral causes of plague — heat, insects, rats — but only *one common cause, the plague bacillus,* so there are uncounted peripheral causes of cancer — tar, radiation, arsenic, pressure, urethane, sand — but only *one common cause of cancer,* to which all other causes lead, the irreversible damage to respiration.

The irreversible damage to respiration is followed, as the second phase of cancer development, by a long battle of the injured cells for existence, in which a part of the cells die due to energy deficiency, while others succed in replacing the irretrievably lost respiratory energy with glycolytic energy. Because of the morphologic inferiority of glycolytic energy, the highly developed somatic cells are converted throughout into undifferentiated, randomly growing cells — the cancer cells.

Cancer Prevention by Support of Respiration

As a direct consequence of the Warburg theory, support of respiration should make tumor development more difficult. There is a surprising example of this.

In Scandinavia there is found a form of cancer of the pharynx and the esophagus which in its early stages — the so-called Plummer-Vinson syndrome — can be easily diagnosed. If the coenzymes of the respiratory enzymes (nicotinamide, flavin, and iron salts) are added to the diet, this precancerous stage can be completely cured. This means that this form of cancer can be prevented, and in fact people are now working to eliminate it by dietary supplementation. In this case, prophylaxis seems to have no problems, since there is obviously no overdosage of these coenzymes.

In addition to this cancer prevention à la Warburg, a cancer therapy à la Warburg is beginning to develop (pp. 208 ff.) in which glycolysis is utilized.

Not All Tumors Show the Warburg Effect

If glycolysis is the actual cause, the decisive characteristic of a tumor cell, then all tumors must show this behavior. In 1958 the first tumors were discovered that do not show aerobic glycolysis (Aisenberg, Potter). They belonged to the series of minimal deviation hepatomas, transplantable liver tumors which differ only slightly from normal liver. It turned out that there is a connection between the growth rate of such a hepatoma and its degree of glycolysis: rapidly growing tumors showed a clear production of lactic acid, but the slowly growing tumors showed little or no glycolysis.

Burk later also made measurements on these minimal deviation tumors. His experiments are summarized in a curve (Figure 29). In the region of the origin (glycolysis of liver = 1) are found slowly growing hepatomas with very little glycolysis. The form of the curve suggests that glycolysis is very low, but is not lacking completely.

The "zero point" is an object of debate: $Q_M^{N_2}$ for liver is given as 1.0 or 0.6, depending on the author. Thus, a glycolysis value of 1.2 for a slowly growing Morris hepatoma appears to be hardly significantly higher than the value for liver.

The criticism goes deeper than this, however: if cells are maintained under oxygen deficiency for 48 to 72 hours before measuring their respiration, they show a greatly reduced respiration. If these cells are then allowed to grow further in normal air, they can again attain their normal respiratory values. Since low oxygen pressures

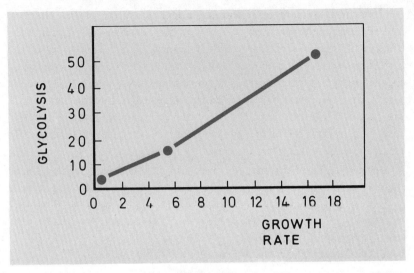

Figure 29

are the rule in most tumors, tumor cells would have to respire at reduced levels anyway, without having suffered from actual damage to respiration.

Many tumor cells do show a "real" injury to respiration; they contain fewer mitochondria and maintain reduced respiration and elevated glycolysis even after extensive periods in air. But it appears questionable whether respiration and glycolysis are also coupled in a reciprocal relationship.

Paul has gone into this question with the system of polyoma-transformed cells. It turned out that the transformed cells did produce more lactic acid, but that they consumed as much oxygen as nontransformed cells. Thus, they are not an exception to the rule of glycolysis in tumor cells, but they also show that a damaged respiration is not obligatory for all tumor cells.

Polyoma-transformed cells are reminiscent of embryonic cells: in these cells, too, the respiration is intact, simultaneously with high glycolysis. In liver regeneration, however, glycolysis is absent. Therefore, growth does not automatically mean elevated glycolysis. Why glycolyzing tumor cells are autonomous and embryonic cells can be regulated must remain unexplained for the moment.

Glycolysis and Growth Rate of a Tumor are Correlated

The series of Morris hepatomas illustrates that slowly growing tumors glycolyze little and that rapidly growing tumors glycolyze much more. The respiration is correspondingly injured and the number of mitchondria reduced.

Burk brought out an analogous finding on tumor cells in vitro. He compared two tumor cell lines which originally derived from the same cell, but which had attained greatly differing malignancies in the meantime. The less malignant line showed minimal glycolysis, the more malignant line showed a high rate of glycolysis.

In a recent investigation of the respiratory and glycolytic enzymes present in normal liver and tumors, Weinhouse found that highly-differentiated minimal deviation hepatomas have the same complement of isoenzymes as normal adult liver, yet these tumors are definitely malignant and will kill their hosts.

Even when glycolysis and growth rate go together, however, this is no proof that glycolysis is the single and possibly solely deciding factor for this growth rate. Why shouldn't glycolysis be the result of neoplastic transformation instead of its cause? To the question as to whether damage to respiration and glycolysis are really primary events in carcinogenesis, Warburg answered that one cannot imagine anything more primary than respiration and glycolysis. Yet the experiments carried out by Weinhouse come close to being the proof that damaged respiration is a product, and not a cause, of tumor formation.

Summary

Damaged respiration and elevated glycolysis of many tumor cells stand at the center of the Warburg cancer theory. Cancer appears to be a relapse into the primitive life customs of the "true" single-celled organisms.

Even if all tumors obviously do not glycolyze, still the growth rate of tumors stands in direct relationship to their degrees of glycolysis.

TUMOR IMMUNOLOGY: BASICS OF A
HOST-SPECIFIC TUMOR DEFENSE

Organ transplants succeed only with art and trickery: to perfect technique by the surgeon must be added outwitting of the host's defense mechanisms. But these are old problems. Van Helmont, a Flemish physician of the seventeenth century, reported:

> A certain resident of Brussels had lost his nose in a battle and went to the famous surgeon Tagliacozzus, who lived in Bologna, with the request to supply him with a new nose. Since he was afraid of having a cut in his own arm, he hired a porter, out of whose arm — after a financial agreement had been reached — a new nose was formed. About 13 months after he had returned home, the transplanted nose suddenly became cold, decayed, and fell off within a few days. His friends, who were interested in an explanation of the reason for this misfortune, found out that the porter had passed on at just the same time that the nose became cold and foul. There are still reputable people in Brussels who were eye witnesses to this story.

Obviously, people believed in predestination at the biological level, in the existence of an inner clock which pitilessly runs down according to predetermined plans. But ignoring this Calvinistic interpretation, van Helmont describes quite exactly what happens when an organ is transplanted into an uncompatible host: at first the organ appears to "take", but then suffers from deficient vascularization — the nose feels cold — it becomes necrotic and ultimatively rejected. The organism recognized the new nose as a foreign body and eliminated it accordingly.

The situation is entirely analogous to the processes after a bacterial infection. Here, too, foreign structures are recognized as such and rendered harmless. Thus, the organism has at its disposal the ability to distinguish between "self" and "nonself." The mechanisms brought to bear in the service of this xenophobia are very complicated: plasma cells, lymphocytes, spleen and lymph nodes, in short, the entire reticuloendothelial system is involved. A complete series of tactics is available: production of neutralizing, agglutinating, and precipitating antibodies, killing by direct contact between cells, phagocytosis, etc. Most of these immunological modes of reaction are highly specific. An antigen fits only on *its* antibody, as a key in a lock. It is inconsequential whether antigen and antibody are soluble or bound to cells. It is conveniently unnecessary to have an overview of the entire immune system and to be acquainted with all its partial functions, if one wants to understand the basic experiments of modern tumor immunology. People are currently inclined to the idea that rejection of transplants and battling of bacterial infections are only "part-time jobs" of the immune system. Transplantations are surely very artificial situations, and we must take into account the fact that the rejection reaction simply makes use of a mechanism originally "thought up" for an entirely different purpose in the organism. "There is an insistent suggestion," Burnet once proposed, "that immunological self-recognition is derived from the processes by which morphological and functional integrity is maintained in large and long-lived multicellular organisms."

The actual assignment of the immune system would thus seem to lie in control of the inner equilibrium of all cells in the whole organism. A special, but highly important, function within the scope of the assignment is the elimination of tumor cells. Just such a host-specific "garbage disposal system" is at the center of the recently revitalized tumor immunology.

Donor-Recipient Relationships in Transplantations

Without additional aids, transplantations succeed only when the donor and the recipient are monozygotic twins. Fortunately, this situation can be approached very closely in animal experiments, by using highly inbred strains. These are strains that have been maintained for an extensive period exclusively by brother-sister mating, and in which, after a few years, essentially all of the animals are genetically identical. They have the same chromosomes and thus not only look alike, but are alike even down to individual protein structures. This case is shown in Figure 30 and is characterized by the terms *isologous* or *syngenic*.

In all other cases (again see Figure 30), exchange transplants are rejected, between animals of different strains *(homologous)* as well as between animals of a not especially inbred strain, and naturally between animals of different kinds *(heterologous)*. The rejection of transplants between genetically different animals (homologous transplantation, "homograft") has been thoroughly investigated. The genes responsible for *histo-incompatibility* could be analyzed. These genes

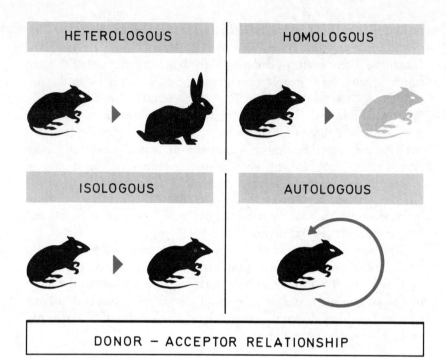

DONOR – ACCEPTOR RELATIONSHIP

Figure 30

regulate the production of substances which differ from one animal to another, except when they are identical twins. These substances are antigenically active — they evoke rejection reaction by the immune system — and thus bear the somewhat pompous name histo(in)compatibility antigens.

How does it happen that transplants from donors with the same heredity are tolerated, and that others are rejected? The question can be put this way: why doesn't the organism's immune system react against its own structures and substances? What keeps the organism from destroying itself? The old immunologists spoke of a "horror autotoxicus," but only modern theories — primarily associated with the names Burnet and Lederberg — gave a clear answer. According to these proposals ("clonal selection theory"), a very young animal possesses a large number of immunologically competent cells, that is, such cells as can make specific antibodies against certain substances and structures. Now, all the cells that can make antibodies against substances in their own organism first react with these substances, are then somehow sensitized, and thereafter drop out of the picture. In this manner, those immunity cells that can react with structures belonging to the body are removed. The other immunity cells are left over, those that have not found a partner, and among them are always some that can later enter into a reaction with foreign substances. Thus, young animals become "tolerant" to antigens peculiar to their bodies and simultaneously to those from donors with the same inheritance. The iron-clad rule that transplantation can take place only between animals of like inheritance thus finds a clear explanation.

This rule recognizes a remarkable exception: spontaneous and experimentally induced tumors can also be transplanted between animals of different heredity. Of course, this succeeds only in rare cases, but in the course of time more transplantable tumors have been found, and there is now available a rich offering of such inoculable tumors.

Transplantable Tumors

Transplantation of tumors was successful even in the last decades of the nineteenth century. Tumors from dogs could be transplanted into young dogs (Novinsky 1877); Moreau passed a mammary gland carcinoma of the mouse (1889). These transplantations were even continued through several passages. In each case, histomorphological investigation showed that the newly grown tumors were identical with the inoculated material. Successful transplantation was thus assured.

These experiments had already shown — to be confirmed in uncounted later experiments — that cancer is transferable by living, intact cells of the body. In transplantation, tumor cells are grafted to the organism, in complete analogy with the work of a gardener who transplants parts of a plant onto another one. For a long time it remained incontestable dogma that intact cells are an undismissable precondition for the transplantation of tumors. Only in the era of virus tumors did this dogma slowly fade away. Today many tumors are known which can be transplanted by cell-free extract.

But these theoretical aspects were not the only contribution of the transplantation pioneers. They had opened up for the first time the possibility of producing tumors ad libitum. People were thus relieved of the necessity of waiting for spontaneous tumors.

At first this early work went almost unnoticed. Shortly after 1900, however, Loeb and Jensen again took up transplantation experiments, and within a few years people everywhere began to study inoculable tumors. Only small pieces of tumor or a tumor brei were needed, dispersed with some physiological saline, and injected with a syringe: beneath the skin, into a muscle, or even into the peritoneal cavity. The first golden age of cancer research had dawned, and people were convinced that the riddle of cancer would shortly be solved. "Cancer is in principle a curable disease," wrote Gaylord in 1906 in a report to the commissioner of health of the state of New York. He based his optimism on the discovery that mice which had healed spontaneously from a Jensen implantable tumor could not be successfully inoculated a second time: they had become resistant. It was now hoped that it was simply necessary to study these "natural" defense mechanisms to arrive at a useful tumor therapy.

Early Hopes for a Protective Injection Against Tumors

Gaylord's mice had become spontaneously cured and thus become resistant. This resistance could also be artificially induced. It was only necessary to preimmunize the animals — either by injections of "subthreshold" numbers of tumor cells, by the surgical removal of an already present tumor, or by the injection of radiation-killed cells. Ehrlich was able to immunize his mice against all of the transplantable breast cancers available to him. These "immune" animals could still, however, die from their own breast cancer. It turned out more and more in the course of time that transplantable tumors are difficult to compare with spontaneous tumors. They metastasize much more rarely and are easier to influence with radiation and medication. Inoculated tumors remain "foreign bodies" that have been forced on their hosts. Any tumor therapy thus comes up against the defense mechanisms which were there all the time. Medawar could consequently come up with the biting remark that "in the study of transplantable tumors you can learn a lot about transplantation, but not much about tumors."

There seemed to be a fundamental change in the situation when people began to work with pure inbred strains. In these animals of common inheritance, transplantable tumors should no longer react as foreign bodies. In fact, isologously transplanted tumors were 4 to 5 times harder to kill with X-rays than homologous transplants. In this respect they are entirely analogous to primary tumors, so that the opinion arose that tumors in genetically identical animals offer a better model for spontaneous tumors. However, all attempts to protect genetically identical animals against later transplantation by preimmunization foundered at first. The idea was already being considered that such measures were doomed to failure, just because of the identity of genetic constitution. Why should a tumor from a monozygotic twin behave differently from a skin transplant from a monozygotic twin? Such a skin transplant is not rejected either.

Tumor-Specific Antigens in Genetically Identical Animals

In 1953, Foley succeeded in showing that defense mechanisms are also mobilized against transplantable tumors in genetically identical recipients. In 1957 his experiments were confirmed and extended by Prehn and Main. These authors first induced a fibrosarcoma in a highly inbred mouse by implantation of a grain of methylcholanthrene. After this primary tumor had grown, they transplanted small pieces of this tumor into a number of other animals of the same inbred strain. These pieces grew and developed into daughter tumors. The latter were then removed and the "cured" animals inoculated a second time with the same tumor. This time the tumors did not grow. Obviously during growth of the first transplant there had come into play defense mechanisms which prevented a "take" of the second transplant (Figure 31 — read down the left side — summarizes the protocol). The operated animals had thus become "immune," even though the tumor came from a genetically identical animal and should not have evoked a defense reaction. We must conclude that the tumor possessed one or more new antigens foreign to the otherwise genetically identical animal, and which therefore induced a rejection reaction. A tumor from an identical twin does behave differently from a simple skin transplant.

Transplantation followed by an operation was not the only method for producing "immune" animals. In many cases a preimmunization was used, with tumor cells killed by a high dose of X-radiation. These suspensions of dead tumor cells also evoke immune reactions which then block the growth of live cells from the same tumor.

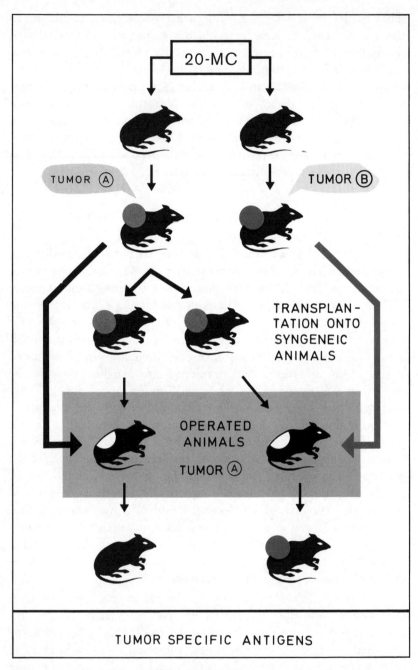

Figure 31

The existence of tumor-specific antigens is not restricted to methylcholanthrene sarcomas. Entirely similar results were obtained with sarcomas induced with other carcinogenic hydrocarbons. Hepatomas induced by azo dyes also showed tumor-specific antigens, as did mammary carcinomas induced by methylcholanthrene. Even sarcomas arising from implantation of cellophane proved to be antigenic, although only weakly so.

Immune Animals Can Only Handle a Few Cells

The transplantation of small pieces of tumor is a relatively crude method. A refined procedure uses instead tumor cell suspensions with exactly known cell counts. It turned out that it can be very important not to inject too many cells, if the second transplant is to be rejected. Even 4×10^5 cells per animal can already be too many.

This could explain the numerous failures of previous attempts: people had usually injected too many tumor cells. The immune system had been simply overtaxed.

The Defense Against Tumor Cells Can be Pretransferred to a Test Tube

In processes which eventually lead to rejection of a transplanted tumor, the lymphocytes surely play a key role. Even without the help of soluble antibodies, lymphocytes can specifically inactivate tumor cells. Direct contact between an "immune" lymphocyte and a tumor target cell appears to be necessary and sufficient.

These reactions can be carried out in a test tube (Figure 32). A few cells from a tumor line maintained in culture were injected into a mouse. After a few days immunologically active lymphocytes could be isolated from the spleen of the immunized animal. These lymphocytes were mixed with tumor cells and incubated at $37\,^{\circ}C$; after 6–9 hours the lymphocytes had killed off the tumor cells. The death of the tumor cells could be elegantly demonstrated with the following method: the tumor cells were labeled with radioactive ^{51}Cr, before the reaction with the lymphocytes, by simply being incubated a short while in a chromium-containing solution. When the labeled tumor cells are now lysed by the lymphocytes, radioactive chromium is released. One only needs to centrifuge down the unlysed

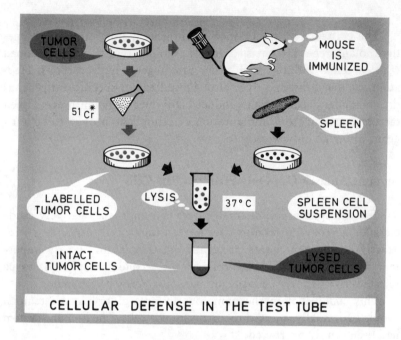

Figure 32

cells: the amount of chromium found in the supernatant then shows how many cells were lysed.

If tumor cells which have been incubated with active lymphocytes are back-transplanted into an animal, this transplantation fails: the defense against these tumor cells had been pretransferred to the test tube.

Individual Tumors Have Individual Antigens

Prehn and Main had found that the different sarcomas which they had induced with methylcholanthrene all possessed differing tumor-specific antigens. If a series of animals had been immunized against fibrosarcoma A — by pretreatment with radiation-killed cells or by other methods — then these animals were immune only against tumor A. Other tumors (B, C...) could grow unhindered in these animals (Figure 31). Conversely, tumor A grew without difficulty in animals which had been immunized against other tumors. It even turned out that tumors which appeared simultaneously in the same animal can have different tumor-specific antigens.

132

After numerous separate investigations it was found more and more that *antigenic individuality of single tumors is characteristic of chemically induced tumors.* Naturally, it should not be expected that all chemically induced tumors would each have to have an individual characteristic antigen. Certainly there will be cross reactions, i. e., animals immunized against tumor A will be immune against some other Tumor X. This would then mean that the antigens specific for tumor A are identical with or closely related to those of tumor X. Such cross reactions have in fact been observed, although only rarely.

Virus-Induced Tumors Also Have Tumor-Specific Antigens

It can be shown, using the same methods as those for demonstrating tumor-specific antigens in chemically induced tumors, that virus tumors also have such antigens. But there is a decisive difference from the chemically induced tumors: all tumors evoked by one and the same tumor virus contain the same antigen. The same virus always induces the same antigen, regardless of whether the tumor grows in a mouse or a hamster. Even human cells maintained in culture form the same antigen, after infection with a tumor virus, as is characteristic for tumors of this virus in hamsters and mice. Thus, the monstrous variety of antigens from chemically induced tumors is in stark contrast with the monotonous group specificity of virus tumors.

The virus tumor antigens have nothing to do with the actual virus particle; they are not, for example, components of the protein coat of the virus, at least as far as DNA tumor viruses are concerned. If one prepares antibodies to the virus itself, they do not react with whole tumor cells. Thus, the virus tumor antigens are a cell product produced as a response to the infection by the virus. What it is that programs this cell product, the genome of the cell itself or the genome of the virus, has not yet been decided. Very probably the virus genome is responsible, for otherwise it would be difficult to understand how the same antigen can be formed after virus infection of very different cells.

Tumor-Specific Antigens Evoke a True Immune Reaction

We have called those animals "immune," in which syngenic tumor transplants did not take, after appropriate immunization. This nomenclature assumes that it was really the immune system of the animals that was responsible for protection. There are several reasons speaking for a true immunological defense.

The high specificity of the reactions by itself indicates the immune system: tumor A induces immunity only against itself, not against other tumors. It is just this strict exclusion that is characteristic for immunological reactions. A patient who has just had scarlet fever can easily get diphtheria, and recovery from flu is not much help against polio. Besides this, there are indirect indications that the rejection of tumor transplants in genetically identical animals really is based on an immune response.

The Rejection of Syngenic Tumor Transplants as a Model for Defense Against Primary Tumors

Modern tumor immunology appears to many to be a "study of interesting artifacts," and a weighty objection is immediately obvious: the transplantation of tumors — even in genetically identical animals — is a highly artificial situation. At first sight the spontaneous or chemical induction of a tumor has very little if anything to do with transplantation.

But let us assume that the immune system of a higher organism really does play a role in maintaining equilibrium with single organs and groups of cells. Then the immune system could play a central role in defense against primary tumors: it would be directed against all cells which "were not around" when the system learned to distinguish between self and nonself. All cells that did not yet belong to the organism when the immune system took shape would be considered foreign. This would mean that all tumor cells, too, which newly appeared in the life span of an organism would have to be automatically categorized as foreign.

Now the question of whither a cell is "foreign" or "nonforeign" to an organism can be answered by a transplantation experiment. If the transplant grows, it was not foreign; if it is rejected, it was recognized as foreign. Considered in this way, the transfer of a tumor into an immunized genetically identical twin does not appear as pure artifact. The recipient twin recognizes the tumor as foreign to just the same extent as the donor, for both of them have the same complement of body cells.

The experimenter makes use of two tricks and no more:

1. he enhances the immune reaction of the recipients before the tumor implantation (preinoculation with the same tumor, which is then surgically removed; preinoculation with killed tumor cells, and the like)

2. he holds the cell count low enough for the preimmunized animal to have a chance to handle the tumor cells.

The original tumor bearer, from which the transplant was obtained, obviously could not hold its tumor in check. In spite of that, there are indications that even this animal had felt its tumor to be foreign. Therefore, let us next look at an experiment which shows that tumor-specific antigens are not only "new" for other animals of the same inbred strain, but also for the primary tumor-bearing animal.

A Rat can Mobilize Defenses Against its Own Primary Tumor

The mobilization of defenses in the primary host can be shown in an experiment very similar to the previously described attempts to immunize several animals (Alexander). 3,4-Benzpyrene was implanted under the skin of a rat; after 8 months a primary sarcoma developed. This tumor was surgically removed and used for preparation of a cell suspension. As a control to establish that there were intact, living cells in the suspension, 2×10^6 cells were injected into genetically identical animals.

Tumors developed in all the animals. When the same number of cells was back-transplanted into the original host, however, tumors developed in only 10 percent of the cases (i. e., the attempt to transfer the primary tumor back into its original host had to be done ten times before a tumor finally took). The hosts accordingly must have possessed defenses that offered extensive protection against back-transplantation of their own tumors.

One question comes up immediately: why did the tumor then grow in spite of these defenses? Obviously there is a quantitative problem involved.

This is shown in a slightly modified experiment. This time part of the primary tumor was allowed to remain in the host. Then 2×10^6 cells per "partial-tumor-bearer" were back-transplanted, exactly as before. This time there were takes in 70 percent of the cases. The defense against the transplanted tumor cells had obviously been extensively "used up" by the residue of the primary tumor. Here again, immune defense against primary tumors is shown to be only limited protection. When too many cells must be held in check, it has to give up. In fact, host-specific immune defense is not only a quite limited defense against tumor cells, it can obviously collapse completely.

In order to understand this collapse, let us consider a modern method which permits the demonstration of killing of tumor cells by lymphocytes of a cancer patient (Hellström): tumor cells are isolated from a tumor and seeded in small numbers in miniature plastic culture dishes. They grow, divide, and after 4 to 8 days form colonies which can be easily counted (Figure 33). Now, if tumor cells which have just begun to grow are treated with lymphocytes from the same host from which the tumor cells were obtained, a few of these cells are killed by the lymphocytes. Hence, fewer colonies are obtained, and from the decrease one can evaluate the immune defense of the host ("colony inhibition test").

With this technique it could again be shown that many tumor patients possess lymphocytes which attack their tumors. Beyond this,

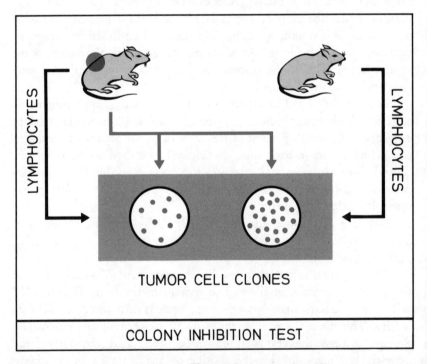

Figure 33

however, this technique supplied a surprising explanation of why lymphocytes chafing at the bit in fact often do not attack. If the tumor cells in the plastic dishes are treated not only with lymphocytes from the host, but additionally with host serum, they grow almost undisturbed into colonies: the serum blocks the effect of the lymphocytes on the tumor cells ("blocking factors").

Thus today we can give (at least) two explanations for the growth of a tumor despite immune defense:

1. The number of immune cells is insufficient to kill all the tumor cells.

2. The immune cells are neutralized by "blocking factors" and can no longer attack.

Do Tumor-Specific Antigens Necessarily Belong to Tumor Growth?

Tumor-specific antigens are widely distributed. In many cases, to be sure, the rejection reaction which can be evoked by tumors is only weak. This is true for the spontaneous mous adenoma investigated by Riggins or for the sarcomas (more closely analyzed by Klein) that grew after cellophane implants. In numerous spontaneous tumors it has not even been possible to show any antigenicity at all.

Accordingly the crucial question is: are tumor-specific antigens necessarily part of the equipment of a tumor cell? Of course, the answer cannot be an unequivocal yes. It would be hard to understand why many tumors obviously have hardly any antigens of this type, or none at all, if these antigens are really decisively important for the properties of a tumor cell. In the case of these antigens, it is easier to think of them as being a consequence of the progression to malignancy rather than as a cause of these malignant properties, a consequence that does not always have to take place. But this view would also be hasty.

The same carcinogen can induce tumors with entirely different degrees of antigenicity. "Early" tumors are more strongly antigenic than "late," with "early" meaning a short latent period, and "late" a long latent period. Late tumors — it can be interpreted — have been filtered through the immune system longer, through a system which can remove tumor cells more easily if they are more antigenic. We must probably draw the conclusion that tumor cells can gradually lose antigenic structures which were newly developed at the beginning of progression.

Even with transplantation tumors, the experience had been noted again, that they become increasingly dedifferentiated ("simplified"), including increasing rubbing off of their antigenic properties. Tumors that could be transplanted originally only within a very limited sphere of recipients can finally be transplanted over a broad spectrum of animals. We could thus hold to the concept that tumor-specific antigens are a necessary part of the initial equipment of a tumor cell. When they are lacking, one would conclude that they have been lost again.

But why should they necessarily be part of the start-up equipment? Today a participation of the surface structures of the cell is being contemplated in growth regulation. Tumor cells — which have largely escaped growth regulation — have also altered cell membranes (see page 98), and it is thus imaginable that the decisive changes in a tumor cell, as compared with a normal cell, are just these changes in cell membranes. Altered cell surfaces would have a twofold consequence: on the one hand they would give the cell the possibility of escaping the regulatory forces of the organism; on the other hand, however, altered surface patterns would mean the same as altered antigenicity. But then the new antigens would necessarily be coupled with cancerization.

Are there Really Tumor-Specific Antigens?

It seems a bit late to ask this question. It is worth considering however that tumor-specific antigens were defined solely by transplantation reactions. A positive transplant rejection test was taken to signify the presence of new antigens. In this sense, but only in this sense, we can say for now that these antigens exist.

This does not mean that someone will not be able someday to isolate these antigens as single substances and characterize them. The chances are not all that great, to be sure. At least there has been very little success up to now in evoking an immune reaction with cell extracts instead of with whole cells. Whenever an immunization was achieved, it was considerably worse than a whole-cell immunization. In the preparation of cell extracts, the cell membranes and most of their fine structure are destroyed. And it probably depends on these membranes and their fine structure.

Cell membranes, i. e., the cell surfaces are surely important for immunological recognition of a cell. Not only because the cell surface can be easily imagined to be the "face" of the cell, but also because cell surfaces have to be able to have mutual recognition in the reactions between tumor cells and lymphocytes. Complementary structures come under consideration as recognition signals: negative charges on the lymphocytes would correspond to positive charges on the tumor cell; protruding structural components of the tumor cell would correspond to depressions in the lymphocytes.

As already mentioned, tumor cells have altered membranes relative to normal cells. But transplantation experiments detect just these membrane changes. Changed fine structures offer new, foreign antigen structures, not tolerated by the immune system. It is not necessary that individual building blocks of the cell surface actually change. Simple changes in complementary arrangement, changes in neighboring relationships would suffice to create new antigen structures. It would also be enough if a certain building block were lacking, in order to get a new grouping in the mosaic of the remaining pieces. New antigenic groups could then arise in great numbers. According to this conception, tumor-specific antigens appear to be missing positions, "holes" in complex structures, rather than variations in an antigen basic substance or a variety of chemically comprehensible new building blocks. The question of whether tumor-specific antigens really exist, would thus possibly be answered "no" by the analytical biochemist.

It would then have to be an electron microscopist, in a position to observe the cell surfaces, who would make visible the "antigens" concluded to exist from transplantation experiments.

Antilymphocytic Serum Promotes Tumor Growth

Immunosuppressives have become medications in great demand after Barnard's heart transplants. They must hinder rejection of the transplanted organs. Cytotoxic substances and cortisone derivatives have been used, but primarily antilymphocytic serum. This antiserum — prepared by immunizing horses or rabbits with lymphocytes — appears to be the method of choice, theoretically: it avoids the cell damage of cytotoxic immunosuppressives and also the side effects of extensive hormone treatment. Despite this, antilymphocytic serum is not without problems, for one cannot cripple the immune system very long without problems. Not only because the danger of infectious disease is heightened, but primarily because the defense against primary tumor cells is endangered.

In any case it has been shown with all clarity in animal experiments that antilymphocytic serum hastens the development of tumors or facilitates the formation of metastases. These experiments are a quite clear indication that immune processes are important in the appearance of a tumor. In concrete terms, a tumor cell is in constant danger of being recognized by the immune system and wiped out. Thus, it is by no means "art for art's sake" to pursue tumor immunology.

Chemical Carcinogens are Immunosuppressives

25 years ago Haddow showed that there is a clear parallel between the carcinogenicity of a substance and its cytotoxic effect. In most cases it proved to be that good carcinogens were also highly toxic for cells. In the meantime it has been found that cytotoxic substances also frequently block the immune system. A large number of the immunosuppressives now used in transplant surgery are further developments of medications that had originally been applied as cytotoxic substances in tumor therapy. It could thus be expected that cytotoxic carcinogens impair the immune system, and in fact an extensive parallelism between carcinogenic and immunosuppressive activity was found. The more carcinogenic a substance, the more it hindered rejection of skin transplants (as an example).

Such transplantations are quite involved experiments, and thus simpler methods were sought for analyzing the functioning capability of the immune defense under the influence of carcinogens. Stjernswaerd used sheep erythrocytes. If these cells are injected into a rat, the animal forms antibodies against sheep erythrocytes within a few days, synthesized by lymph cells in the spleen. These cells can be isolated and mixed with fresh sheep erythrocytes in agar. In the gelatinous mixture the cells remain immobilized and thus only the immediately neighboring red blood cells are effected when the lymphocytes release their antibodies. When complementarity is present, the antibodies lyse the erythrocytes, and after a short time there are clearly recognizable halos in the colored erythrocyte layer. These "plaques" can be easily counted and form a direct measure of the number of antibody-producing lymphocytes (Jerne test; Figure 34).

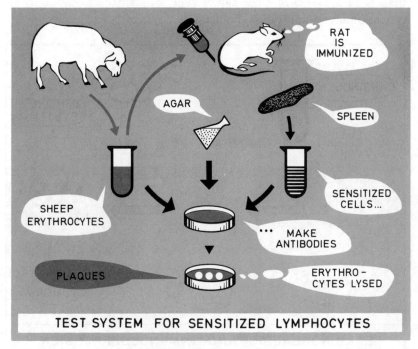

Figure 34

Using this test, Stjernswaerd analyzed the immune capacity of rats after, say, the subcutaneous injection of 0.5 mg of 3-methyl-cholanthrene, a quantity sufficient to induce malignant sarcomas after a few months. It turned out that the immune capacity was considerably reduced throughout the entire latent period. These analyses also showed, therefore, that chemical carcinogens act as immunosuppressives and that even at the low doses which are sufficient to produce tumors, they can have an effect on the immune defense system.

Nothing is said by this as to whether the reduced defenses have an influence on tumor development, but it would not be very easy to see why the immunosuppressive effect of antilymphocytic serum should be important for tumor formation, while the immunosuppressive effect of chemical carcinogens should have no significance.

The Double Effect of Chemical Carcinogens

Thus, a carcinogen could carry out two functions: it effects the transformation of normal cells into tumor cells, and it increases the chances of survival of these tumor cells, by damage to the immune system (immunosuppression, Figure 35).

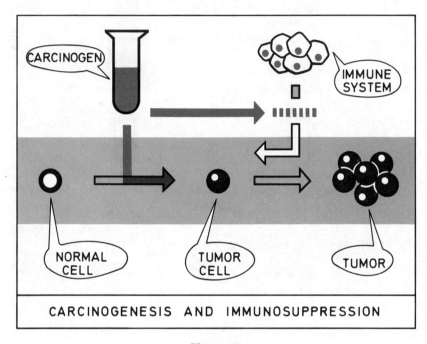

CARCINOGENESIS AND IMMUNOSUPPRESSION

Figure 35

A further possibility appears conceivable. If there were potential tumor cells to begin with in a living organism, which simply are not expressed because they are constantly being swallowed up by the immune system, then the immunosuppressive effect of the carcinogens could be their actual carcinogenic effect — their actual mechanism of action.

This would have a very gloomy consequence: all biochemical investigations on carcinogen-treated tissues would then be nothing more than studies of the toxic effects of carcinogenic substances; they would have nothing to do with the actual carcinogenesis. This would then take place in the complicated network of the immune defense mechanisms, far from the target cells under investigation.

Immune Therapy

The old dream of being able to immunize against cancer has at least come true in part. Mice and chickens have been successfully immunized against tumor viruses and were resistant from then on against leukemia viruses. Immunological protection against chemical tumors really ought to be impossible, for the variety of possible tumor antigens prohibits the preparation of a generally effective immunity agent. Here we are theoretically not much farther than Ehrlich got with his breast cancer in mice.

More important than prophylactic measures with their limited scope of applicability are those attempts to combat gross tumors immunologically. These efforts can be divided into three groups: 1) unspecific stimulation of the immune mechanisms of the host, 2) active immunization, and finally, 3) passive immunization.

1. The normal immune defenses of a tumor host are low. The transplantation experiments on "immune" animals have shown that mice can combat only a few million cells; solid tumors contain many more cells, by several orders of magnitude. But even in 1924, Murphy was able to greatly reduce the appearance of spontaneous metastases after surgical tumor removal, by stimulating the immune defense system with oleic acid. In 1964 this experiment was repeated by Martin, although with less sensational results than Murphy had. (He used Zymosan to stimulate the immune system.) The repeated injection of the Bacillus Calmette-Guerin (BCG) also strengthens the rejection reaction against transplants. The same treatment also led to regressions of tumors. Most recently Poly I/C has been used as an immunostimulant.

The methods for unspecifically winding up the body's own immune reactions are still somewhat in a stage of alchemistic unclarity. To be sure, the methods of transplantation research permit directed maneuvers, but by and large there is a lack of established concepts. In contrast there are clear ideas at the basis of attempts to immunize specifically, with passive as well as active methods.

2. It is conceivable that a growing tumor only releases a few cells and that consequently the immune response of the host is not running at full throttle. In such a case, a postimmunization with the same tumor would exploit the residual capacity of the reticuloendothelial system. In a case studied by Haddow and Alexander, it was found that tumor regressions were observed if the immune system had been

"heated up" by the injection of cells from the same tumor. To be sure, a local treatment with X-rays was also required.

3. The immunity against tumor transplants can probably be ascribed predominantly to immune active lymphocytes. This knowledge makes possible a direct *passive* immunization of the host. The tumor from the animal to be cured is transplanted to other syngenic animals, resulting in the initiation of an immune reaction against these tumors. "Immune lymphocytes" can then be obtained (spleen, thoracic duct) and injected into the original tumor bearer.

Enhancement: The Paradoxical Increase in Tumor Growth by Immunization

If animals are immunized with killed tumor cells, the chances that a tumor transplant takes and grows are diminished, as we have discussed. Occasionally, however, just the opposite effect occurs: the tumor grows faster if the animal has been preimmunized with tumor material.

This enhancement appears to depend on a mechanism other than the induction of a tumor immunity. Animals that have been made immune against tumors have lymphocytes that are active against the tumor cells. Animals that have been enhanced have soluble antibodies also directed against the tumor cells. The differences emerge clearly if one in one case incubates tumor cells with lymphocytes and in another case with antibodies of an immunized animal: in the one case (after treatment with hymphocytes) the tumor cells are killed and do not grow in the animal; in the other case (after antibody treatment) there is accelerated cell growth. If we want to explain the phenomenon of enhancement, we can start from the idea that the soluble antibodies occupy the antigenic structures of the tumor cells. Two consequences are then possible:

1. The overlaid tumor cells cannot release any further immune reactions which would have led to the induction of active lymphocytes.

2. The overlaid tumor cells can no longer be attacked by lymphocytes, since the regions on the cell surface necessary for identification by the lymphocytes have been covered up and become unapproachable.

In both cases the normal reaction of immune lymphocytes against tumor cells has been hindered; surveillance of the tumor cells has consequently been disturbed, and the tumor can grow without interference.

Enhancement is the Damocletian sword of immunological therapy of tumors. As long as it cannot be predicted with certainty whether a procedure will lead to immunity or enhancement, all immunological measures for inhibiting tumor growth can be overturned into the opposite: instead of the hoped-for destruction of the tumor, the tumor growth is increased.

Summary

The discovery of tumor-specific transplantation antigens indicated the existence of a tumor surveillance system in the body of the host. Chemically induced tumor A immunizes its host against a second transplantation of the same tumor, assuming sufficiently low cell numbers. High cell counts in transplantation can easily overrun the barriers set up by immunization. Immunization with chemically induced tumors is highly specific: tumors other than the one used for immunization can generally be transplanted without "resistance."

In contrast, tumor-specific antigens in virus tumors are the same in all tumors induced by a given (DNA) virus. They are not identical with the antigens of the virus particle itself.

Antilymphocytic serum hastens tumor growth; possibly the immunosuppressive "side effect" of chemical carcinogens plays a role in carcinogenesis.

The immunotherapy of tumors uses measures to activate the immune defense systems. Active and also passive immunizations, together with classical therapeutic methods, have led to tumor regressions. Unspecific activation of the immune system can also be used therapeutically.

Occasionally, increased tumor growth results paradoxically from immunization with tumor material: this phenomenon of enhancement is a serious fly in the ointment for all immunotherapeutic endeavors.

NATURAL HISTORY OF SOME TUMOR VIRUSES

"Cancer is not an infectious disease." Hundreds of years of experience by surgeons and pathologists had graven this sentence in stone;

precautionary measures had never been taken in handling tumor material, and had never proved to be necessary. The cancer ward is not an isolation ward. It must have seemed a ridiculous idea to propose in all seriousness that viruses can occasionally cause cancer. Viruses are responsible for smallpox and influenza epidemics, but what should they have to do with stomach carcinomas and lung cancer?

But, virus research had always been a revolutionary science. The first Dutch virologist, Martius Willem Beijerinck (1851–1931), a botanist by profession, shocked his colleagues with the announcement that he had succeeded in transplanting tobacco mosaic with cell-free extracts from diseased plants. Beijerinck had purified his extracts over thick filters which had retained all bacterial cells for certain. But bacterial cells were an absolute requirement for infection according to all bacteriologists; "cell-free extracts" could not possibly be infectious.

Thus, the first virologists were simply scorned; people maintained that they either had holes in their filters or holes in their heads. Patiently Beijerinck wrote: "The existence of these contagions proves that life — if metabolism and reproduction are considered its most important characteristics — does not have to be inseparable from structures. In its most primitive form life is like fire and is nourished like a flame by living substance; a flame that does not arise from generation out of nothing, but is passed on by other flames." One would speak of "fire and water" in the language of the old theory of elements.

The blockheaded Dutchman also had privately revolutionary ideas. When he was appointed to the Delft Polytechnical School, he had a discussion with the director about reorganization problems. When the director indicated that the administration must continue to exist, Beijerinck countered: "If anything has to go, it is the position of director." Problems of this type are still discussed; Beijerinck's theory about "fluid life" was quickly discredited, however.

It was soon recognized that even the "filterable viruses" have a definite size, and the particles could even be measured, using calibrated filters. Viruses could not, however, be cultivated on artificial media. Virus reproduction does not take place without living cells. The slogan "borrowed life" or the designations "parasite at the intracellular level" and "vagabond genes" characterize the situation. Viruses compel the host cell to supply energy and material for the production of new viruses. When the viruses have taken over command, the cell works against its own interest on this assignment. A virus-infected cell is marked by death, and a virus without a cell is actually dead.

When Stanley discovered that the tobacco mosaic virus (TMV) can be crystallized, the viruses appeared to fall completely out of the realm of biology. Today the excitement over "crystalline life" has largely died down, and virus research has become a solid member of the biological establishment.

The tumor viruses had to fight longer for recognition. From the very beginning, tumor viruses seemed to be in direct contradiction of two basic dogmas of medicine:

1. They obviously disregarded Virchow's concept of cancer as a cellular and only a cellular disease. According to Virchow's conception, the cancer cell became a cancer cell "on its own"; a parasite was not consulted.

2. They occasionally, however, set themselves above Koch's postulates.

Robert Koch had demanded, and all bacteriologists still do, that the cause of an infectious disease is only known after a whole series of requirements has been fulfilled:

a) The microorganism must be demonstrated in each and every case of disease. Microscope and agar dish are the most important tools.

b) The causative agent must be *susceptible to cultivation* in pure culture.

c) These pure cultures must be able to induce the disease in suitable animals.

d) The agent must also be isolable from the newly diseased animal and capable of being further cultured.

Koch himself and many others since have proceeded according to these strict rules and thus identified the stimulants of numerous infectious diseases. Pasteur, in contrast, already had to skimp a little: to be sure, he could transfer the "rabies agent" from one dog to another and even from rabbit to rabbit. But he could not see the "virus" or culture it outside a living organism.

The tumor virologists got into even greater difficulties. They, too, could neither see their "tumor-agents" under the microscope nor succeed in getting them to multiply in artificial media. But even worse was the fact that often they could not even isolate anymore virus from the tumors they had induced with cell free extracts: the virus seemed to have disappeared from these tumors. Often neither could characteristic virus particles be detected in these tumor cells, nor was there any success in preparing infectious extracts from virus tumors. For this situation the virologists coined the term "masked virus."

In reality, however, the viruses had not disappeared at all: first traces were found, and finally the masked viruses themselves. Viruses can do more than just crudely flail out; they do not always have to force the host to produce one virus particle after the other to the point of self-destruction. A cell can very well survive a virus infection, but occasionally at a high price: it can lose the ability to fit into a higher organism. It becomes a tumor cell, and thus finally kills its host organism and itself as a consequence.

Let us first present the most important representatives in a short natural history of tumor viruses.

Chicken Leukemias

Chronic leukemias are not a rare disease in chickens. The bone marrow and lymphoid organs such as the spleen or the lymph nodes are attacked. In addition, chickens can suffer from a "red leukemia," in which immature erythrocytes (erythroblasts) take over in the blood picture.

In 1908 the Danes Ellermann and Bang found that such *erythroblastoses* can be transplanted cellfree. The "filterable agents" are present in diseased chickens in such quantities that a nanoliter of blood suffices to infect a healthy chicken.

The history of tumor viruses should have been able to begin with this discovery, but at that time leukemias were by no means recognized as "cancerous diseases." The dogma of the exclusively cellular nature of cancer thus remained undisturbed for the moment.

Besides these erythroblastoses in chickens, there also occur *myeloid leukemias*. This form is also induced by a virus and can be transferred in cell-free extract. Unfortunately, chickens have extreme variability in their reactions to these viruses, even when they are of the same strain. Large numbers of animals were therefore necessary to get statistically certain results. J. W. Beard and D. Beard have consequently had to develop outright assembly line methods to deal with these difficulties. There was no problem whatsoever in getting enough virus: 1 ml of blood can contain a billion infectious virus particles. Simple ultracentrifugation is enough to concentrate these particles.

In contrast, the *lymphatic leukemia* of chickens could for a long time not be passed. This was especially annoying because of the great economic significance of this form of leukemia. In places where fowl breeding is done on a large scale in limited quarters, almost half of the flock can be attacked by this disease. Lymphatic leukemia had become a kind of "cultural disease" of chickens.

In this form of leukemia the leukemic blood cells usually get "stuck" in the tissues and do not float out into the bloodstream ("aleukemic form"). Tumor nodules are found primarily in the greatly enlarged liver, but also in the lung, the pancreas, the kidneys, and even in the skin.

Successful transfer of lymphomatous tissue was not accomplished until 1941, and five years later Burmester and coworkers (USDA Poultry Research Laboratory, East Lansing, Michigan) reported the first successful cell-free passage. Another ten years later the first vaccines were available. The first protective injection against cancer was a reality. The fact that "only" a virus tumor was involved somewhat took the sheen off the joy of victory.

Large scale investigations were undertaken in East Lansing to find out how this lymphomatosis spreads. Two pathways were found:

1. This form of leukemia can be transmitted via the egg to the offspring (so-called "congenital" or "vertical" infection — Figure 36).

2. Direct infection was also observed: if chickens from a "healthy" strain were mixed with "sick" animals, the healthy animals also came down with lymphomatosis. A closer analysis showed that transfer was through the air, but that only very young animals could be infected ("horizontal" infection).

Thus, chicken lymphomatosis bears features of a classical virus disease, be it an epidemic influenza or a trivial sniffle. "Wouldn't it be interesting, if other tumor viruses would spread like a simple cold?," asked R. J. Huebner of the National Institutes of Health. Interesting, certainly, but highly unsettling.

Careful investigations, however, have never really indicated that human tumors could be infectious. Such investigations are monstrously difficult from the start, because very long latent periods after a successful "infection" have to be reckoned with, before a tumor can be diagnosed. Clear recollections here are probably rarely possible. If decades were to pass after infection with a sniffles virus, before the

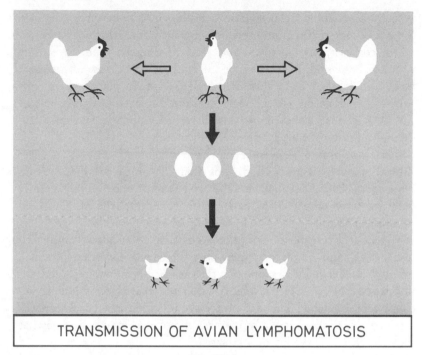

TRANSMISSION OF AVIAN LYMPHOMATOSIS

Figure 36

sniffles broke out, a clear etiology of the disease would be practically impossible.

Rous Sarcoma Virus (RSV)

Tumor virus number one is without doubt the Rous sarcoma virus. There had been lively discussions as to whether the chicken leukoses were really true cancers. For a solid sarcoma, however, the diagnosis of whether it is a tumor or not is considerably easier.

Peyton Rous, a young pathologist at The Rockefeller University, was the first to succeed at cell-free transplantation of a spontaneous chicken sarcoma (1910). He had prepared an extract from a sarcoma in the breast of a Plymouth Rock hen, purified it through bacterial filters, and finally injected it into the breasts of young chickens of the same breed. In a few of these animals there developed tumors which metastasized to the lungs, liver, and other organs in the same manner as the original tumor. Thus, Rous was certain that he had induced true tumors with his extract. There could be no doubt that a virus was involved. Still Rous was cautious and quite undeceitfully named his sarcoma virus a "tumor agent." In spite of this, hardly any notice was taken, and the high priests of cellular pathology refused to accept it: it takes more than one virus to make a believer in "cell-free cancer."

In fact there were difficulties again and again in cell-free passages. The cell-free preparations were usually low in viruses, which meant that inoculation at best resulted in poor yields, if none at all. "Tumors rich in virus are entirely an artificial product of the laboratory," even Oberling, an enthusiastic advocate of a general virus etiology of cancer, conceded, "an artificial form obtained by continuous passaging in very young animals over an extended period of time."

Shope Papilloma Virus in Rabbits

Wart-like growths have long been noticed again and again in the cottontail rabbit of Kansas and Iowa. Many of the warts were so large that hunters spoke of "horns."

In the early 1930's R. E. Shope had tried to transmit such tumors cell-free. The tumors were pulverized, filtered, and the filtrate rubbed into domestic rabbits after the skin had been scraped with sandpaper. The first papillomas appeared after about a week.

Wild rabbits could also be infected with these extracts, but there were important differences (Figure 37):

1. In *wild* rabbits the tumors grow slowly and as a rule lead to large horny warts ("papillomas"). These tumors can be rubbed off mechanically, and spontaneous cures are even possible this way. In *domestic* rabbits the papillomas grow faster and become less horny than in the wild rabbits.

2. The virus itself also behaves differently in the domestic and wild rabbits. Viruses are demonstrated in the slowly growing papillomas of the *wild* rabbits, by electron microscopy and by further infection with cell-free extracts. The tumor in the *domestic* rabbits do not contain any free virus. Extracts from these tumors do not induce tumors in other rabbits.

Thus, no one would presume that the tumors of the domestic rabbit are virus tumors. Even though induced by a virus, the virus has disappeared in the gross tumor. Of course, they have not disappeared without a trace. Here we refer to a masked virus. What this means in molecular biological terms will be covered later in more detail.

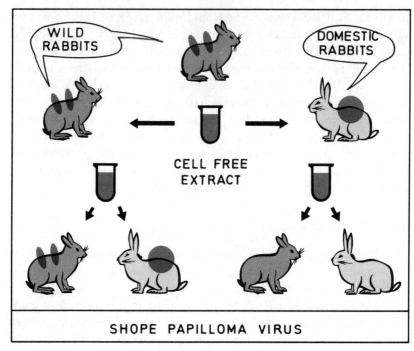

Bittner's Milk Factor

There are strains of mice with a high incidence of mammary tumors, and strains with essentially none. When such strains were crossed, there was great surprise: it was by no means immaterial which of the parents was derived from a breast cancer strain. The offspring succumbed to breast cancer much more frequently when the mother was from a tumor strain. This stands in contradiction to Mendel's laws, and investigators started to wonder whether the inheritance of cancer could be connected with extra chromosomal factors.

In 1936, Bittner found a simple explanation: the mother's milk contains a factor that promotes breast cancer. If young mice from a mammary tumor strain are brought into the world by Caesarian section and suckled on "wet nurses" from a tumor-free strain, then the young mice do not later develop breast cancer. They have therefore forgotten their "genetic" disposition to breast cancer. The reciprocal experiment was equally successful: young mice from a tumor-free strain developed mammary tumors if they were suckled by "tumor wet nurses". Bittner called his factor the "milk-borne mammary tumor agent" and stuck to this neutral designation even after people recognized that a virus must be involved (cell-free transmission, multiplication in sensitive animals, isolation of virus particles with the ultracentrifuge, electron microscopic detection).

But quite soon it was found that a virus alone is not enough to induce breast cancer in these mice. The Bittner factor is effective only in certain strains. Here we see the significance of genetic disposition, of a strain-specific sensitivity of the mammary gland cells. Besides this, mammary carcinomas can only arise when the mouse is in a favorable hormonal state: if the ovaries of the mice are removed, thus stopping a large part of the production of female sex hormones, then no breast cancer occurs.

In summary we can say that the Bittner virus can induce mammary carcinoma if there is a certain genetic complementarity and assuming that enough female hormone is present. Beyond this, the age of the mouse cannot be ignored: infection directly after birth leads to later tumors in 100 percent of all cases; the tumor incidence is reduced to 60 or even 10 percent, if 20-day-old or 120-day-old mice, respectively, are infected. These complications are naturally encountered only when the animals have *not* been infected by the mother's milk.

The mice sicken only when all factors "agree." "It is surely time that we should drop medieval concepts concerning causation and think in terms of multiple correlation," Julian Huxley has written, and the Bittner case clearly illustrates this thought.

Polyoma

Mouse leukemias can also be transmitted cellfree. In 1951, L. Gross was able to prepare a cell-free extract from organs of leukemic mice, which again induced leukemia in newborn mice.

Sarah Stewart repeated the experiments and could also transmit mouse leukemias. To her surprise, however, leukemia did not arise in an inbred strain. Instead there developed in these mice after 10 months tumors of the parotid gland and the adrenal gland. Then there came the usual letdown: active cell-free extracts could not be prepared from the parotid tumors. Here, too, the tumor-inducing virus had disappeared again.

She then collaborated with B. E. Eddy of the National Institutes of Health. Eddy had built up a large productive tissue culture laboratory in which a large part of the work had been done which eventually led to a polio vaccine. Monkey kidney cells had been shown to be an ideal "nutrient medium" for the polio virus.

Stewart and Eddy now attempted to reproduce the new "parotid virus" on such kidney cells. The results were extremely meager: as before, the tumor yields were low. Perhaps the problem was that a mouse virus does not multiply well in monkey cells. Hence, Stewart tried again in mouse cell cultures. Mouse embryos were carefully minced and trypsinized into single cells. The cell suspensions were then inoculated into culture bottles and the consequent cell layers treated with organ extract from leukemic mice.

Now the virus showed its true colors: cell-free preparations from these infected mouse embryo cells induced malignant tumors in almost 100 percent of the animals treated. But the unambiguous result was not the only remarkable part. The virus-enriched extracts did not produce just parotid tumors any more:

> The thymus gland, an organ just above the heart, was frequently involved; in many instances a tumor of this organ filled the chest cavity. Contradicting the rule that tumors of the mammary glands develop only in female mice, the virus engendered cancers in the mammary glands of males as well. Tumors of the lungs were usually of the type that involves the mesothelium, the outer covering of the organ, and they covered the entire lung with fingerlike projections that could be seen with the naked eye. Cancers of the skin often covered the entire body surface. The sweat glands, present only in the hairless surfaces of the mouse foot, also developed tumors. All of these are cancers of the epithelial type and are classified as carcinomas. But the virus also induced sarcomas: cancers of connective tissue, bone, kidney, the lining of blood vessels and the cysts of the liver. We even found a tumor in nerve tissue that arose from the virus (Stewart).

The massive doses had permitted recognition of an astonishing virulence. Occasionally as many as 10 different types of tumors were found in a single mouse. Hence, the discoverers gave their new virus the name "polyoma" — the many tumor inducer.

But was it really only one virus? Wasn't it just as probable that a whole virus family was involved? If different viruses were involved, then one would expect that upon virus production in tissue culture, some would reproduce better than others. Then after many, many passages certain of the viruses would die out while others got the upper hand. But after almost 100 passages in tissue culture, the virus preparation still induced the same variety of tumors. It was therefore concluded that "polyoma" does not represent a mixture of different viruses with different target organs. This conclusion was finally confirmed with "genetically pure" strains of polyoma (strains derived from a single virus particle). Every single pure culture of polyoma which was investigated again produced the same multiplicity of tumors as the original virus preparations.

Polyoma had still more surprises in store. The tumor viruses known up to that point were very choosy in their choice of host. The Bittner virus grows only in certain strains of mice. But the polyoma virus crossed the barriers between mouse strains with ease, and even those between species: polyoma induces tumors in hamsters, rats, and rabbits. Hamsters proved to be especially sensitive: tumors appear after only 2 weeks.

But why hadn't people ever run across polyoma virus in nature? The skeptics were again able to claim that virus tumors are simple artificial products of the laboratory. But there are "natural" explanations.

Polyoma virions are excellent antigens. There are antibodies in the blood of inoculated animals directed specifically against this virus, regardless of whether the animals got tumors or not. Even animals that merely sat in the same box with virus-treated mice had produced antibodies in many cases. Nor does polyoma have any respect for man: a few coworkers in the Stewart group who had worked for years with this virus also had polyoma-specific antibodies.

In mouse colonies the virus is spread via saliva and excrement. Mouse mothers can pass on polyoma antibodies to their offspring, however, so that spontaneous polyoma tumors are rare. Only in tissue culture, when there are no antibodies, can large amounts of polyoma be prepared.

Mouse Leukemia and Mouse Sarcoma Viruses

We have already mentioned: mouse leukemias can be transmitted cellfree in the same manner as chicken leukemias. There is a whole series of different virus strains, named after their discoverers: Gross, 1951; Friend, 1957; Rauscher, 1962.

Sachs has described a simple quantitative assay for the Rauscher virus: a dilute virus solution is injected into the tail vein of adult mice. After about 9 days, clearly visible nodules are formed in the spleen, which can be easily counted.

These mouse leukemia viruses are related to the leukosis viruses of fowl (the Rous sarcoma and the recently discovered mouse sarcoma viruses also belong to this family). There are immunological and morphological family similarities.

1. These viruses have common (group-specific) antigens.

2. They have characteristic forms in the electron microscope (dark nuclei with a somewhat removed outer coat); the so-called C-particles are in this family.

Using this immunological-morphological "wanted poster," RNA tumor viruses have been demonstrated recently in cats, hamsters, and dogs. Occasionally C-particles were even found in human cells.

Human Medical Digression

For a long time, warts have been the only (benign) new growths in humans with an established viral etiology. (The wart virus is related to the Shope papilloma virus.)

Human leukemias primarily stand under strong suspicion. However, direct proof has been lacking. Granted, C-particles could be found again and again with the electron microscope, but the proof that these particles had also caused tumors is naturally impossible. Still, the chain of evidence grows stronger. After all, why should C-particles cause leukemias in chickens, mice, and cats, and not in humans? A recent piece of evidence revealed by Gallo and coworkers is the discovery in human acute lymphoblastic leukemia cells of an enzyme which: 1) is not found in normal human lymphocytes, and 2) appears to be a characteristic for RNA tumor viruses. (See the end of the next chapter for a more complete discussion.)

In the last few years the so-called Burkitt's lymphoma was recognized as the "first" human virus tumor. A malignant lymphoma of the neck and jawbone is involved, which frequently appears in certain regions (equatorial Africa). Epidemiological, immunological, and electron microscopic analyses have made a virus of the Herpes group responsible. A similar virus appears to induce the long-known so-called Lucke kidney tumor in frogs.

What will be the next "human" tumorvirus? There is no lack of candidates, and human breast cancer has been under suspicion for a long time already. Here it is not necessary to first embark on a long search for viruses; they have already been found, even in the milk. They are similar to the Bittner mouse factor: they belong to the so-called B-particles and posses the enzyme reverse transcriptase, as do many other RNA viruses (see p. 176). In addition, it appeared that there was an increased incidence of virus in women with a family history of breast cancer (Moore). Spiegelman, finally, could show that in breast tumors it is often possible to demonstrate the presence of a RNA with a base sequence like that of the Bittner factor. All of these findings led Spiegelman to the remark: "If a woman has a history of breast cancer in her family and if she shows (milk) virus and if she was my sister, I would tell her not to nurse the child."

This is consistent thinking, for Bittner had been able to show that in mice the mammary tumor virus can be transferred via the milk. In mice it is sufficient, therefore, to have the mouse babies nursed by a virus-free wetnurse, in order to avoid breast cancer. In man there seem to be much more complicated relationships, summarized as follows: "There has been a huge decrease in breast feeding over the past 30 to 40 years and if anything there has been a slight increase in breast cancer (Shubik)". In the meantime Moore had discovered that not only B-particles are present in mother's milk, but also C-particles in particular. Even more, significant differences between "history" and "non-history" women could not be confirmed, and the authors conclude that these viruses obviously are quite widespread. But to conclude from this that viruses do not play a role in human breast cancer would be most negligent. The clear cause and effect relationships that Bittner could demonstrate in his mice are veiled in humans by all too many distorting factors (genetic, hormonal, dietary, environmental, social).

Human and Monkey Viruses: Adenoviruses and SV-40

Monkey kidney cells in large quantities are used in the preparation of polio vaccine. A monkey virus was discovered in such cultures, which evoked tumors in newborn hamsters. (SV-40 denotes a certain type of such a Simian Virus.) As yet no human disease is known which could have something to do with SV-40; but people have been careful to avoid contamination of polio vaccine with this virus.

SV-40 can also transform tissue culture cells into abnormal, "tumor-like" forms. This transformation proceeds not only with hamster cells, but also with human cells. If such transformed hamster cells are implanted into young hamsters, they grow into tumors. Experiments with human SV-40–transformed cells are naturally out of the question.

But SV-40 did not remain the only tumor-inducing primate virus. Trivial human cold viruses proved to be oncogenic. These adenoviruses were first isolated from the adenoids of infected children. They were encountered again and again during cold epidemics. In recruits, especially, exposed without protection to new viruses in a new environment, the viruses cause painful throat inflammations.

If they are injected into newborn hamsters, adenoviruses can cause tumors. Not all adeno types are oncogenic: Adeno 12 (out of about 30) is an example of a type that does cause tumors.

Classification of Animal Viruses

Obviously, there are no basic differences between tumor viruses and the "classical" viruses. The classification of viruses can follow several methods (Figure 38, Table 5).

RNA or DNA: Generally a virus consists of a "nucleus" of nucleic acid and a "coat" of protein. One speaks of DNA or RNA viruses accordingly.

Helical or cubic: The individual building blocks of the protein coat can be orientated "cubically" or in a spiral: the classic example of a helical virus is TMV, which to be sure does not belong to the animal viruses. Cubic "virus crystals" in contrast are polyoma or adenovirus. The DNA is within the "crystal," and the proteins are arranged on the edges of an icosahedron.

With or without coat: The basic virus (nucleic acid + protein coat) may or may not be packed in another coat. Frequently, a part of this coat consists of components of the cell membrane. The virus helix is occasionally coiled to fit better in such a coat.

Large or small: Finally, viruses can be classified simply by size, and people speak of "small DNA viruses" such as polyoma or SV-40.

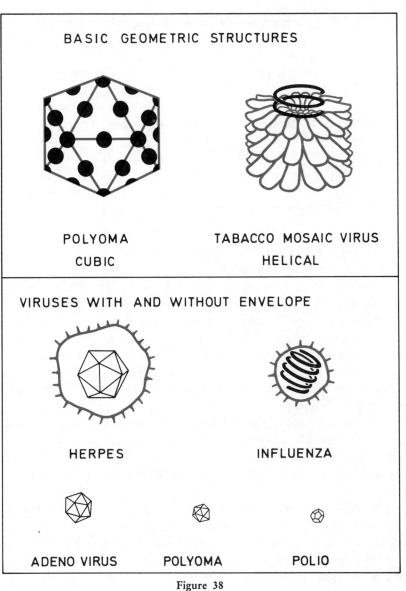

BASIC GEOMETRIC STRUCTURES

POLYOMA
CUBIC

TABACCO MOSAIC VIRUS
HELICAL

VIRUSES WITH AND WITHOUT ENVELOPE

HERPES

INFLUENZA

ADENO VIRUS   POLYOMA   POLIO

Figure 38

Tumor viruses do not form a special group within such a scheme: the influenza virus is found alongside RSV, and the adenoviruses along with polyoma.

This subdividing goes even further, however. The same virus can pop up as a tumor virus as well as a "classical" virus. A special type

Table 5: Classification of Viruses Pathogenic in Animals

Helical		Cubic		
RNA	DNA with coat	RNA with coat	DNA with coat	DNA without coat
Influenza	Myxoma	Enteroviruses	Herpes	Adenoviruses
Mouse leukemia	Pox	Reoviruses		Polyoma
Bittner milk factor	Shope fibroma	Polio		Shope papilloma
Avian leukosis				SV-40
Rous sarcoma				Adeno 12
				Warts (human)

of the "sore-throat virus" — Adenovirus 12 — is definitely carcinogenic: when it is injected into newborn hamsters, metastasizing sarcomas form within a short time.

The dual identity is shown especially clearly by influenza virus: mice that are treated with this virus get an influenza-like disease. If they are treated with tobacco smoke, nothing happens. But if the mice are subjected to tobacco smoke and influenza virus simultaneously, they get lung tumors (Leuchtenberger). A "harmless" virus thus becomes a tumor virus, in combination with "harmless" tobacco smoke. This clearly shows that "classical" viruses can "turn over" into tumor viruses.

The reverse phenomenon is also widespread: occasionally tumor viruses behave like normal viruses. In very young animals a tumor virus can cause cell destruction and consequent hemorrhages. This has been observed with the Shope papilloma virus and the Rous sarcoma virus.

We will tentatively conclude that the decision as to whether a certain virus induces a tumor depends considerably on the target cell. But let us put off a deeper discussion of this question and turn first to the behavior of viruses in tissue culture. We are limiting ourselves for reasons of space to the small DNA viruses polyoma and SV-40.

Summary

Cancer research was not part of the triumphal march of bacteriology at the turn of the century: all attempts to implicate a bacterium in the induction of animal tumors foundered. Germs that had been isolated from tumor tissue always turned out to be harmless fellow travelers or secondary infections. Hence, the tumor viruses were looked at with the greatest mistrust; but in the course of time, numerous oncogenic viruses have elbowed their way into the arsenal of tumor-inducing factors.

Tumors of very different kinds can be induced by viruses: skin tumors (Shope papilloma virus), kidney carcinomas (polyoma), mammary carcinomas (Bittner milk factor), and many others. At the top of the heap are sarcomas (Rous sarcoma virus) and leukemias of all varieties in chickens, mice, and, recently, cats.

Tumor viruses are not basically different from the viruses that are "classical" pathogens in animals: the leukosis viruses are in the same group as the influenza virus. Viruses of the same type can have an oncogenic as well as a "classic" (cell-killing) effect: certain types of the adenoviruses that cause sore throats cause tumors in newborn hamsters.

Tumor viruses can go underground: tumors induced by viruses need not always contain viruses. As an example, the Shope papilloma virus has "disappeared" from the rapidly growing papillomas of the domestic rabbit.

DNA TUMOR VIRUSES IN TISSUE CULTURE

More and more tumor viruses were discovered; ever more tumors could be induced by viruses. But for a long time tumor virology was in a precarious position.

In many cases strict proof was lacking that the tumors were really virus tumors, for from many virus-induced tumors the virus had disappeared. The classical criteria of bacteriology therefore had to fail when applied to virus etiology.

The methodological problems were often just as precarious: rapid experiments were made impossible by latent periods running from several months to over a year. Exact experiments remained wishful thinking: many experimental animals had widely varying reactions to virus preparations, and the virus preparations themselves differed greatly in activity from charge to charge.

There was a basic change in this state of affairs when the techniques of tissue culture were applied to problems of tumor virus research: "Certain tumor viruses readily multiply in these cultures, allowing accurate quantitation and efficient production of virus, but sometimes they cause a transformation of the normal cell to one having the properties of a tumor cell. And all this can be demonstrated not in months, but in as little as a few days!" (Habel).

Before we turn to the behavior of DNA tumor viruses in tissue culture, we have to clear up a practical problem.

Counting Live Viruses in the Plaque Test

Viruses can be counted directly under the electron microscope, but dead viruses and "empty coats" are also included, easily leading to false conclusions. Hence it makes more sense to count only the active particles. For this one must find a cell type in which the virus reproduces well (monkey kidney cells for polio, mouse embryo cells for polyoma), inoculate these cells into a petri dish, and wait until a dense cell layer has grown. Then the cells are inoculated with a dilute virus solution, the virus is allowed to enter the cells, and the culture is layered over with agar. This trick prevents virus particles freed by

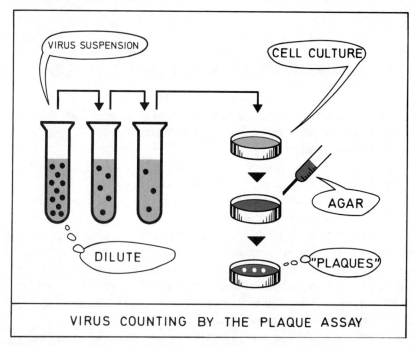

VIRUS COUNTING BY THE PLAQUE ASSAY

Figure 39

lysis of infected cells from unhindered diffusion. Hence they can only infect the respective neighboring cells and, again only there can they reproduce. In this manner a single virus eats, as it were, a hole (plaque) in the cell layer visible with the naked eye. If the virus solution to be tested has only a few *virions* (plural of individual virus particles), the few holes appearing on the plate cannot run together. They can then be easily counted, and thus one obtains a measure of the number of active virus particles — "plaque-forming units," PFU, "infectious" (see Figure 39).

Many viruses pathogenic in animals can be quantitatively determined in this manner: polio viruses, adenoviruses, and tumor viruses, too.

Transformation in Vitro

As a rule, tumor viruses can do more than just punch holes in a suitable cell layer. They can annul strict social rules of a tissue culture.

Many cells also submit to order when in culture. They divide only as long as they have room. If the cell layer has grown dense, cell division stops; the close contact of cell to cell hinders new mitoses ("contact inhibition").

Cells that have been infected with tumor viruses occasionally fail to abide by these agreements: they grow over and on top of their neighbors and form irregular piles. These morphological characteristics alone already bear a distant resemblance to small tumors. It has in fact been proved that these piled-up cells are really tumor cells. If they are implanted into an appropriate recipient (an animal of the same inbred strain from which the culture cells were originally de-

---

How can a transformed cell be recognized?

1. Increased growth rate
2. Capability of unlimited passage in tissue culture ("permanent line")
3. Loss of contact inhibition ("piling-up" and "criss-cross")
4. Appearance of virus-specific antigens
5. Tumor formation in immunocompatible animals

rived), they develop into real tumors. These "criss-crossed cells" had thus been transformed into tumor cells by the tumor virus (Figure 40).

Transformation and Cell Death

Transformation and cell damage can accompany each other: if mouse embryo cells are infected with polyoma virus, the characteristic piling-up can be seen next to the transparent plaques.

Cell death and transformation are two such fundamentally different processes that one really ought to assume also that two different virus types would be responsible. This would have a simple consequence: viruses isolated from an individual plaque should only be able to cause plaques, but not transformation.

Experiment showed just the opposite: transformation and cell destruction appeared next to each other again and again, even when the infecting virions had been isolated from an individual plaque. One and the same virus can therefore produce productive infection as well as transformation.

The Cell can Choose between Production and Transformation

The decision as to whether virus production and the accompanying cell destruction, or transformation and formation of a tumor cell will come about, depends largely on the cell. Cell lines are known which are preferably lysed by SV-40, and others which are predominantly transformed (Figure 40).

Not only hereditary properties of the cell are important; the physiological state of a cell influences the decision between transformation and production. Virus transformations work considerably better with growing, dividing cells than with resting, so-called stationary cells. The virus DNA obviously can thread into the cell DNA easier, if this is just replicating. This means that, besides the cell *line*, the *phase* of the cell cycle is important for the decision on transformation and cell death.

The cells are certainly not completely free in their decision: if one gives a large excess of SV-40 to cells which normally only permit transformation (high multiplicity infection), then "forbidden" virus production can take place.

Several thousand virus particles can be produced in one individual productive cell; in contrast, transformed cells appear to contain no virus at all.

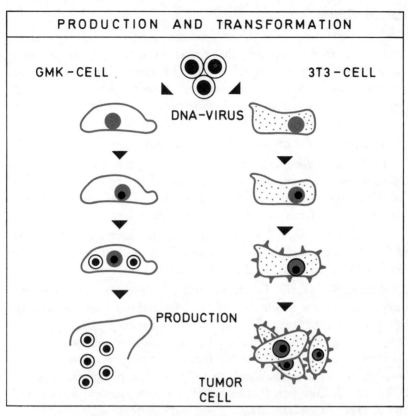

PRODUCTION AND TRANSFORMATION

GMK–CELL

DNA–VIRUS

3T3–CELL

PRODUCTION

TUMOR
CELL

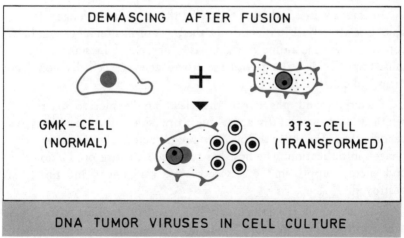

DEMASCING   AFTER FUSION

GMK–CELL
(NORMAL)

3T3–CELL
(TRANSFORMED)

DNA TUMOR VIRUSES IN CELL CULTURE

Figure 40

Masked Viruses

It is not really surprising that transformed cells contain no more virus. This finding corresponds to the old observation that often no virus is demonstrable in virus-induced tumors. (Thus the rapidly growing Shope papilloma in domestic rabbits no longer contains Shope virus.)

Two possibilities are available for explanation:

1. The one possibility is trivial and purports that viruses did indeed cause the transformation, but that they are then dispensable for the finished tumor cell. Accordingly, the viruses would not only have disappeared, but would actually have been lost.

2. But it was soon learned that although the tumor viruses can seemingly disappear, they are not lost. They duck into the cell and live in a "masked form" in the underground.

Bacteriophages are the classic model for such "masked viruses." Phages are viruses which multiply in bacteria and lyse the bacterial cell. But reproduction and lysis do not always take place. There are "mute infections," in which the phage gets into the cell, but does not destroy it. The offspring of such infected bacterial cells are apparently healthy, but they can suddenly, wildly produce phage particles and be destroyed. Different factors set off these delayed explosions: UV and X-rays, peroxides, different dyes, and different carcinogens.

In latently infected bacterial cells, the virus is no longer detectable, but after lysis it is suddenly there again in numerous complete copies. In the meantime it must have hibernated in some form; it must have divided along with the crowd at every cell division. The virus had behaved like a gene.

Bacterium and phage can thus lead an "explosive marriage," which at some time falls apart due to outside influences: the virus genome then takes over the business and is exclusively concerned with phage multiplication. The host has to place its entire production line and energy supply in the service of this assignment and finally is destroyed.

The model of the latent phages is crudely applicable to DNA tumor viruses. Polyoma and SV-40 also do not disappear completely from the transformed cells. Even in apparently virus-free tumor cells, "fresh tracks" indicate the presence of a virus.

On the Trail of Masked Tumor Viruses: Virus-Specific Antigens

The first traces could be found with immunological methods: there are antigens in virus-transformed cells which are lacking in normal cells. These antigens differ according to the transforming virus: thus there are polyoma-specific and SV-40-specific antigens.

Such virus-specific antigens were discovered in the *nucleus* of transformed cells, and were called T-antigens (tumor antigens). Hamsters carrying polyoma-induced tumors produce antibodies against polyoma-specific nuclear antigen. If these antibodies are marked with fluorescent dyes, the antigens can be identified under the microscope: cells with T-antigen display brightly fluorescing nuclei after incubation with labeled antibodies. Cells without antigens remain dark.

The T-antigen is not a component of the virus, such as a protein from the protein coat. Its function is still unclear. Recent investigations have shown that there are virus-induced tumor cells which do not have a T-antigen. Accordingly, this antigen may be unnecessary for transformation.

Virus-specific antigens are also localized on the cell membranes of transformed cells (TRA-transplantation rejection antigens). These antigens are responsible for rejection of transplanted virus tumors. As we saw in the preceding chapter, it is possible to induce a limited degree of immunity against transplanted virus tumors. If one tries to inoculate the same virus tumor a second time into such resistant animals, the transplanted tumor cells do not take, provided that not too many have been transplanted.

The localization of these transplantation antigens on the cell membrane is well established:

1. It is generally assumed that transplantation antigens sit on the cell surface. Only in this way is a direct reaction possible between transplanted cell and defending immune cell.

2. Immune reactions can also be evoked with cell ghosts instead of with intact transformed cells. These ghosts are the outer membranes of cells burst in hypotonic salt solution, but with extensive preservation of the surface substances of the original cell.

Antigenic substances of the virus particle itself (protein subunits) are not identical with the TRA-antigen either. The TRA-antigens are produced by the transformed cell under direction from the virus.

Different types of cells produce the same antigen when transformed by the same virus (see page 133).

In addition to the surface antigens which can be detected by transplantation, there are also those which can be demonstrated directly in the test tube (agglutination test, fluorescein-marked antibodies). These antigens are often designated S-antigens.

Now let us inquire into the biological significance of the transplantation antigens. Transplantations and the rejection of transplants are quite artificial situations, biologically exceptional cases, so to speak, which can only be realized in experiments. Still, there are good indications that virus-specific substances of the transplantation antigen type also play a role in the "normal" developmental history of a viral tumor.

The altered antigenic structures of the tumor cell warn the immune defense system of the host. The transformed cells are viewed as "new" and "foreign" and set off defense mechanisms. The virus has "alienated" some of the body's own cells. This alienation obviously has two effects:

1. The alienated cell drops out of the organizational system of the whole organism; it is no longer subjected to the rules of the society, and thus becomes a tumor cell.

2. It is just this alienation, however, which gives the host a handle with which to reject the tumor cells as foreign material.

According to this concept, the S-antigens are at the center of viral tumorigenesis: the more these antigens alienate a cell, the easier they can escape normal regulatory signals. But they are also more greatly endangered by the immune defense of the body. This relationship is clear, but as yet has not been proved by hard experimental facts.

Virus-specific antigens have not remained the only "fingerprints" of tumor viruses in transformed cells. Virus-specific ribonucleic acids have proved to be especially revealing tracks.

On the Trail of Masked DNA Tumor Viruses: Virus Specific Ribonucleic Acids

Transformed tumor cells produce virus-specific messenger RNA. Demonstration of this special messenger RNA is done with the so-called DNA-RNA hybridization technique; we have to backtrack a bit to understand this method.

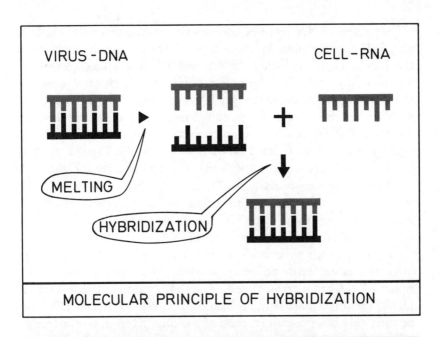

MOLECULAR PRINCIPLE OF HYBRIDIZATION

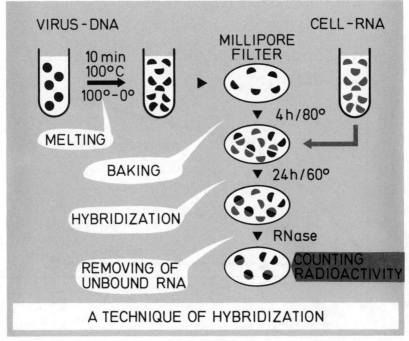

A TECHNIQUE OF HYBRIDIZATION

Figure 41

Messenger RNA receives the genetic information of the DNA, i. e., it is a linear piece-by-piece copy of the nucleotide sequence of the DNA. Hence messenger RNA and DNA are complementary, although any individual messenger only copies a short sequence of the DNA. If DNA and messenger RNA from the same cell are mixed with each other, the corresponding nucleotide sequences line up together. The DNA-RNA complexes can be separated and quantitatively determined. If some DNA is mixed with a random messenger, however, only a slight association is found as a rule (Figure 41).

The information of the virus DNA is also first copied onto RNA molecules, and this virus-specific messenger RNA can also be hybridized with virus DNA. Thus virus-specific m-RNA is defined as an RNA which is hybridizable with virus DNA.

In an attempt to hybridize virus DNA with RNA from non-infected normal cells, no pairing takes place. In contrast, if one isolates RNA from transformed cells and hybridizes this with viral DNA, there is a partial hybridization between RNA and DNA: to be sure, only a very small fraction of the total RNA of a transformed cell can be paired, but the binding to virus DNA is highly significant

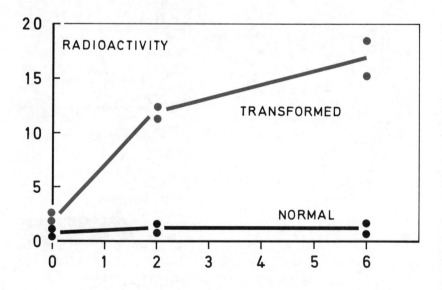

Figure 42

(Figure 42). This means that virus-specific RNA is present even in transformed cells, although the virions themselves are invisible.

This new signpost is a direct indication of the presence of virus DNA, for where would the cell get the information for this RNA otherwise?

Virus DNA is Retained in Transformed Cells

The existence of viral DNA in transformed cells follows not only from the demonstration of virus-specific messenger RNA; but it has also been proved directly.

This proof was again obtained with the pairing technique of complementary DNA and RNA. First, one needs virus messenger RNA as an indicator for virus DNA. This RNA can be isolated from a mixture of cell and virus messengers extracted from infected cells. Westphal chose a more elegant way: he produced SV-40 messenger RNA artificially. To this end he used an enzyme that polymerizes ribonucleotides to polynucleotides (RNA), strictly according to the direction of a so-called primer DNA (DNA dependent RNA polymerase). The sequence of the synthetic RNA is complementary to the sequence of the primer DNA used, and if virus DNA is used as primer, one gets virus-specific RNA.

This synthetic virus messenger RNA now binds to the DNA of a cell transformed by tumor viruses, but not to the DNA of normal cells. It follows that virus DNA is permanently present in the transformed cell. "Masked virus" therefore means nothing but "naked virus DNA," or "nucleus" of the virus particle. Crude estimation indicated the presence of 10-50 virus copies per cell. All copies are localized in the cell nucleus. If we now recall the observation that transformation succeeds better when DNA synthesis is going on in the cells, then we get to the idea that the virus DNA is incorporated into the DNA of the host cell. At each cell division, the virus DNA divides along with the rest. If it did not do that, it would gradually have to be lost, and this has never been observed.

In the strictest sense, the nucleic acid hybridization technique proves only that at least parts of the virus DNA exist in the transformed cell. A new technique now permits the broader conclusion that the entire virus genome of an SV-40 virus can be retained in a transformed cell.

Unmasking of the Tumor Virus: Cell Fusion Forces Virus Production

In the last few years it has become possible to fuse mammalian cells (Ephrussi, Harris). In this process cells form which at first have two or more nuclei. Later a single nucleus is formed, which contains the chromosomes of both "parent" cells.

Such cell fusions between cells of higher organisms are normally rare. They can usually be demonstrated only in special cases, in which the "super cell' formed by fusion has a selective advantage over the simple parent cells. Such a fusion can be brought off, however, by the trick of treating the cells with Sendai virus. This virus — named after a city in Japan — normally causes an influenza-like disease, but can initiate cell fusion in cultures: obviously the virus contains a "fusion factor" which prepares the cell walls for the fusion. This fusion also works with "dead" (UV-inactivated) Sendai virus. This has the considerable advantage of avoiding production of Sendai virus after fusion.

With the Sendai method, Koprowski has fused a whole series of transformed cells (apparently without virus) with normal cells in which virus production can take place. Virus production then started up in the resulting multinuclear cell hybrids. The "productive" cell turns the "masked" virus of the transformed cell into a productive virus (Figure 40).

This experiment proves two things:

1. The entire genome of the virus can also be retained in transformed cells, for after fusion complete virus particles are again produced.

2. Obviously certain reactions do not occur in a transformed cell, which are otherwise necessary for production of complete viruses. There is no synthesis of coat protein and no mass production of viral DNA. A transformed cell holds its virus under control, at least in this respect.

The Virus DNA is Responsible for Transformation

We have seen that transformed cells still contain virus DNA. There is a simple proof that this DNA is also of decisive significance for transformation. This proof was first accomplished with polyoma (Stewart).

Like most other viruses, polyoma can be fractionated into nucleic acid and protein coat. The nucleic acid fraction can then be purified and given to hamster cells. Cells are thereby transformed to tumor cells, exactly as if the cultures had been treated with intact polyoma. Polyoma DNA also proved to be carcinogenic in the whole animal. The conclusion is unequivocal: the nucleic acid of the tumor virus is responsible for transformation.

The tumor virologists have thus confirmed long time experience of virus research: "The nucleic acids are to blame for everything." In 1956 Schramm and Gierer had already demonstrated with tobacco mosaic virus (TMV) that the nucleic acid from TMV can eat the same holes in tobacco leaves as the intact virus rods and that protein extracts from TMV were without effect. In the following years, such "infectious nucleic acids" could be extracted from numerous viruses. If sensitive cells are infected with these infectious nucleic acids, complete virus particles are again produced, exactly as from infection with intact viruses.

Thus the nucleic acids contain all the information needed for a virus to multiply in a cell. Virus DNA and virus genome are identical. The nucleic acid core of a virus corresponds to the chromosomes of a higher organism. In the end, therefore, virus tumors are induced by the genes of the virus.

A DNA Tumor Virus has Only a Few Genes

An "old" theorem of molecular genetics goes: "One gene – one enzyme." What is true for bacteria and fungi also holds for viruses. The genes of a virus also key enzymes and proteins: enzymes which take care of virus multiplication, in addition to those of the host cell; proteins which redirect the metabolism of the cell, and finally proteins which change the properties of the cell membranes.

Let us estimate how many genes are represented by the DNA of a polyoma or SV-40 virus. A single strand of polyoma DNA contains about 5,000 bases, as can be easily calculated from the molecular weight of the intact DNA. From molecular genetics we know that three nucleotides determine any particular amino acid. Thus the total DNA of a polyoma or SV-40 virus can code for about 1,700 amino acids. About a fourth are required to construct the amino acids of the coat protein. The rest would suffice to supply blueprints for about 4 to 8 somewhat small protein molecules. The maximal number of genetic factors which the polyoma virus can bring into a cell would then hardly be more than 5 to 10.

"Since the number of viral genes is small, it should be possible to identify those responsible for cancer induction and to discover how they function in the infected cells" (Dulbecco). First, we must set up a catalog of the known "virus specific events" which take place when a virus has infected a cell.

Which Genes are Suspected of Transformation?

1. After virus infection the DNA synthesis of "resting cells" increases. There is also increased production of the enzymes necessary for DNA replication. Cellular DNA synthesis in a resting cell has stopped. Obviously, then, the viruses are in a position to release this brake, at least partly. Thus this virus function is a good candidate for a function of significance in tumorigenesis.

2. Transformed cells have "new" surface antigens, which are recognizable by transplantation of these tumor cells and by in vitro tests. These antigens are probably coded for by the virus and not by the cell (see page 167).

3. In addition to the transplantation antigens, the nuclei of infected cells have another virus-specific antigen, also not identical with components of the virus particle. It is excluded from the circle of tumor candidates, since some tumor cells have recently been discovered which do not have this T-antigen.

4. The most striking characteristic of a virus is its outer structure, the protein coat. No coat protein is produced in transformed cells, however. These proteins thus appear to be dispensable for transformation. The corresponding gene is thus also excluded as a "tumor-inducing" viral gene.

Only a few further functions can be added to these, but their discussion is beyond our present scope. Thus our catalog shows that most of the possible virus genes have already been discovered. The circle of suspected genes is hence not only small, but is also basically already known.

The first bets have already been made: the virus functions which can induce DNA synthesis are well in the running (see item 1 above). Primarily, however, the surface antigens (see 2), which are recognizable as transplantation antigens, are highly suspicious, since it is they which "alienate" a cell.

Making bets is not quite enough, but the experiments which could bear on a final decision are clear: induce mutation in the individual genes of the virus genome; alternately block all of the functions of the virus in this manner, and see if such a virus is still oncogenic. In this manner it ought to be easy to find out which of these functions is indispensable for transformation.

These experiments appear to be easy, but the short list of only a few genes in the polyoma virus does not necessarily mean that the genetic analysis will be uncomplicated. Individual gene products could enter into complex interactions with each other and thus — in spite of small number of "primitive" genes — lead to a large variety of phenotypic end products.

It has recently been found that the SV virus does not possess only a coat protein; hence, it already now seems certain that the virus genome alone cannot code for all of the known "virus-specific products."

Interactions between cell and virus products are naturally to be expected; here, too, a few virus functions could lead to numerous changes which would all be virus specific. Hence we must discuss the role of the cell in transformation once more.

The Role of the Cell Once More

In the system virus-cell both bear responsibility, and the responsibility of the cell is certainly not small. The same Shope papilloma virus induces rapidly growing, malignant tumors in domestic rabbits, but only slowly-growing benign papillomas in wild rabbits. In very young animals polyoma can lead to cell destruction, without tumors having to appear. The responsibility of the cell is clearest in a few pure cell lines maintained in tissue culture: the hamster cell line BHK and the mouse cells 3T3 can be transformed with SV-40 without any noteworthy virus production. In contrast, virus production is almost the only event in other cell lines.

Hence the cell can determine the type and extent of the infection to a considerable degree. The cell sets the switches that decide whether formation of a tumor cell or virus production takes place. A cell on the way to transformation is obviously in a position to suppress multiplication of a DNA tumor virus.

The control by the cell is radical: the cell forbids translation of the virus DNA into messenger RNA. There is censorship at the level of transcription. Hybridization experiments have shown that less virus information is read in transformed cells than in productive cells. Consequently it can be concluded that it is decided at the level of transcription (DNA → m RNA) whether transformation or production is to follow. Most recently some doubts have been expressed, and it is thought by some that control takes place at the level of translation (RNA → protein) (see page 193).

Thus the cell is responsible for virus production and its own death. Could it also be responsible for transformation?

Let us suppose that each has the potential capability to divide. "Life wants to grow and divide" (Szent-Györgyi). It needs no stimulus, simply a favorable opportunity, Bullough believes: "opportunity cause mitoses." This is surely the case for one-celled organisms, but the cells of a higher organism do not seem to have completely forgotten their primitive state of uncontrolled growth.

According to this concept, a tumor virus only has to trigger a cell to "run away." The virus would simply give a push; the cell can carry on by itself. The functions and characteristics induced by a tumor virus would only have an indirect relationship to the neoplastic properties of a cell or none at all.

The idea that the *virus itself* is in a position to steer the cell on a neoplastic course is of course more fascinating. Then the changes brought about by the virus would more or less directly lead to transformation. At the moment there are no good reasons not to expect this effect from tumor viruses. The solution of the cancer problem would then be in view: it remains to be seen how much time is needed to thoroughly test all the genetic functions of a tumor virus.

A Side Glance at RNA Tumor Viruses

In contrast to the previously discussed DNA tumor viruses, RNA tumor viruses can multiply in infected cells without killing the host. In addition, cells which have been transformed by RNA tumor viruses can still produce viruses. The Rous sarcoma viruses and the leukosis viruses belong to this class.

In tumor cells which were induced by RNA tumor viruses, the membranes are also changed here, and here, too, transplantation antigens were discovered. Thus RNA tumor viruses could "alienate" normal cells in the same way as DNA tumor viruses.

Certain RNA tumor viruses require so-called "helper viruses": only when helper viruses are around can there be virus production. The reason: only these helpers can produce coats; the "actual" tumor viruses finally slip into these helper coats.

RNA tumor viruses had more surprises in store: in 1964 Temin had postulated that these viruses construct a specific DNA according to the base sequence of their RNA, i. e., just the opposite of what normally happens. With this assumption he found it easier to understand (1) that cells which were transformed by RNA tumor viruses remained transformed (transmitted the transformation to daughter cells), and (2) that DNA synthesis must take place as a preface to transformation after virus infection.

If this assumption is correct, then RNA tumor viruses ought to code for an enzyme which polymerizes DNA strands from the virus RNA template. Such a polymerase has actually been discovered (Temin, Baltimore, Spiegelman); it is contained in purified viruses and makes DNA-RNA double strands. Obviously all information does not have to emanate from DNA.

The production of a unique enzyme by these RNA viruses could have tremendous theoretical and medical consequences however, and this fact did not escape other biochemists. Among the consequences imagined was the possibility of using this enzyme as a "fingerprint" for masked RNA viruses. Huebner and others have postulated, with immunological experiments for indirect support, that human sarcomas and leukemias might be caused by masked RNA viruses (C-particles). The discovery of RNA dependent DNA polymerase opened up two possibilities:

1. The presence of a masked RNA virus in a human cancer might be demonstrated.

2. If some human cancers are in fact caused by RNA viruses, the test for the enzyme could serve as a test for early detection of the cancers.

Within six months after Temin's report, Gallo reported that he and his colleagues had demonstrated the presence of the enzyme in human acute lymphoblastic leukemia cells. They further showed that there was none of this enzyme in lymphocytes of normal humans, even after these cells were tricked into going into DNA synthesis.

Meanwhile, Spiegelman's group at Columbia took on the task of establishing the generality of the "reverse transcriptase" presence in RNA tumor viruses. As of August, 1971, this enzyme had been found in almost 30 RNA viruses able to cause cancer in animals.

Thus the RNA tumor viruses could be closely related to the oncogenic DNA viruses, and a "side glance" at these viruses would really be nothing more than a look back at the DNA tumor viruses.

Summary

DNA tumor viruses occasionally lead a double life. In cell culture they can (1) kill the cells (cytopathic effect) or (2) transform the cells. In the latter case, neoplastic cells arise directly, which grow over neighboring cells against the rules of contact inhibition. Tumors arise upon transplantation into suitable animals. The infected cell can influence the choice between production and transformation.

In virus-induced tumors and in transformed cells the viruses can "disappear." Masked tumor viruses are revealed by virus-specific antigens and virus-specific messenger RNA. Thus virus DNA is demonstrable in transformed cells.

A DNA tumor virus (such as polyoma) has only a few genes (fewer than 10). Exact analysis should permit inferences as to what steps are indispensable for transformation. For a tumor virologist the problem of carcinogenesis is reduced "from a problem in cell genetics to a problem of virus genetics. The simplification is one of several orders of magnitude" (Dulbecco).

GENETICS AND CANCER

Virchow's "cellular pathology" had placed the cell at the center of the theory of disease: cells, the bearers of life, are also the seat of diseases. If anyone wants to learn about disease, he must first of all study cells.

Modern pathology did not stop here. Virchow's cells proved to be monstrously complicated structures with their own regulatory organs, energy supply systems, and production plants. These cellular components in themselves are highly complex structures, assembled from many different molecules of the most varying types.

Hence it was entirely logical that the molecular pathology of diseased cells moved on to "diseased molecules" (Pauling). Molecules are "diseased" if, because of some mistake in construction, they are no longer capable of carrying out the jobs assigned to them within the cell and the organism.

The hemoglobins, the molecules responsible for oxygen transport, are a classic example. The substitution of a single amino acid in a peptide chain of hemoglobin by a "wrong" amino acid can lead to a hemoglobin molecule with completely altered properties. Sickle cell anemia is the best known example: in this case, gross morphological examination of the erythrocytes reveals the presence of "defective" hemoglobin molecules. Exact chemical analysis showed that the amino acid valine had simply been replaced by glutamic acid in a peptide chain of the sickle cell hemoglobin.

Often important molecules are not simply changed, but are more or less completely lacking. Here the concept of a "diseased" molecule seems to be inappropriate. But examples of this type of molecular pathology are numerous: diabetes (insulin deficiency), aglobulinemia (lack of globulins), phenylketonuria (lack of enzymes for phenylalanine catabolism), and others. Yet "behind" these missing molecules are again the wrong, "diseased" molecules: deranged enzymes or "mutated" DNA. When people reflected on cancer, they tried here, too, to use of the concept of "diseased molecules." But which molecules were ill in this case?

As a rule, cancer cells give rise to daughter cells which are also cancer cells. This "genetic memory" of a tumor cell can be understood most easily by assuming that the genetic material of the cell is altered. But genetic material means chromosomes means DNA.

The question of which molecule is sick in a cancer cell would then be answered with "DNA." It would probably be better to speak, not of a "diseased" molecule, but of an "unrestrained molecule" (E. Bäumler). This designation clearly characterizes the situation: the reckless division is thus comprehensible as is the transmission of a "craving for freedom" to the daughter cells, for the unrestrained molecule is the genetic material itself.

This idea that chromosomes have something to do with cancer is almost as old as the discovery of chromosomes. Even in the 1890's, people observed altered chromosome patterns and mitotic anomalies in tumor cells, and irregularities in cell division. Theodore Boveri (1862–1915), a biologist in Würzburg, at the beginning of this century formulated his *chromosomal theory of malignant tumors,* summarizing his observations: tumor cells have chromosome numbers deviated from normal.

Chromosome Alterations in Tumor Cells: The Philadelphia Chromosome

Abnormal chromosome numbers have been established again and again in tumor cells. (Diploid and tetraploid cells, as well as cells of higher ploidy all are found, as are chromosome complements in which only a few chromosomes are deficient or in excess.) It turned out that most experimental tumors consist of mixed cell populations with varying chromosome complements, although a certain chromosome grouping ("stem line") is frequently predominant.

Chromosomes altered morphologically can also be demonstrated in tumors. Such marker-chromosomes occasionally facilitate detection and diagnosis of certain tumor cells. The best-known example is the so-called Philadelphia chromosome. It was discovered in patients with chronic myeloid leukemia, and is present in cells of the bone marrow and the blood. Its demonstration permits certain diagnosis. The place of its discovery has been preserved in the name.

The Philadelphia chromosome is an exception. Normally quantitative and qualitative deviations from normal vary from tumor to tumor, from leukemia to leukemia. Since even cells of the "same" tumor can differ in their chromosome complement, cytogenetics (the science of genetic material of an individual cell) has only limited practical value as a diagnostic tool.

Doubts are recurrently expressed as to whether the altered chromosome complements of tumor cells really have anything to do with the special properties of these cells. It would be entirely clear that in cells which rapidly progress from mitosis, more rapidly than they would normally, there would be repeated inexactitude in the sorting out of the individual pairs of chromosomes. The hasty divisions would thus more or less necessarily lead to abnormal chromosome patterns. Chromosomal anomalies would then be simply the result of oncogenesis and not a prerequisite.

If this were so, then there ought to be tumors with fully normal chromosome complements. In the series of the so-called minimal deviation hepatomas, such euploid tumors have actually been determined. Using the usual methods of cytogenetics, no deviations from normal could be established in especially slow-growing hepatomas of this series. This knowledge is hardly new or surprising in human pathology: in human tumors normal chromosome complements seem to be the rule.

Naturally we have not excluded the possibility that submicroscopic alterations exist in the chromosomes, and that these invisible mutations are decisively important for the neoplastic properties of the tumor cell. Geneticists have long sought just such "invisible" chromosomal alterations.

Inheritance Factors in Tumor Induction: Animal Strains with Guaranteed Tumor Incidence

Dr. Maud Slye had a simple working hypothesis: if there is a tumor gene or several, it should be possible to breed these genes into an animal or to breed them out again.

It is basically simple to isolate some property, say a particular color of fur, out of a mixed population. If only those animals are bred that carry this characteristic, one eventually comes out with animals whose entire offspring carries it. The same holds true if one wants to select strains with a high tumor incidence: it is only necessary to reproduce those animals bearing a given tumor. There are considerable problems in breeding pure tumor lines, however. While it is easy to see if a mouse has gray or white hair, in the case of tumor selection one has to wait, possibly throughout the life span of the mouse, until tumors appear. Only then is it known which cross was the right one. All of the offspring obtained in the meantime have to be retained until it is known which ones should be bred further.

Among the more than 200,000 mice of her "mouse house," Maud Slye could see practically all of the tumors known to human pathology. Many of her strains reached 100 percent incidence of leukemia, lung cancer, mammary carcinomas, or other forms of cancer. All of these animals got tumors spontaneously without external treatment, once they had grown old enough. Thus it was proven that cancer is heritable. However, the existence of a cancer gene, in which Slye had believed, became more improbable in the meantime. Today tumor geneticists agree that the induction of a cancer depends not on one, but on many factors.

Let us recall the Bittner factor and breast cancer in mice. There both the virus and the genetic constitution of the mouse were important. But what is meant by genetic constitution in this case? Certain surface properties of the cells, which facilitate virus entry, could be meant. A sufficiently high estrogen level also should be considered, which means that synthesis and breakdown of the female sex hormones in the ovarian follicles and the liver have to be adjusted to each other. But genetic constitution is certainly not sufficiently described in this manner. The more we learn, the more factors we can implicate, and today people will surely want to bring up genetically determined immune defense as well.

Or we can consider a recessive heritable disease such as *Xeroderma pigmentosum*. Here an oversensitivity of the skin to light is inherited. In the first few years of life, inflamed areas appear on exposed areas of skin, followed by a type of wart formation and finally by carcinomas. This cancer appears to be a prototype of a hereditary cancer, but in reality only the light sensitivity is inherited and not the cancer as such.

At bottom, however, this holds for all inheritable characteristics, and not just for genetically determined diseases. Only the tendencies are transmitted, and not the finished characteristics. There may occasionally be simple relationships between genotype and phenotype, but as a rule the complicated interaction of numerous genes is necessary to develop complex structures such as an organ or a wing. We should not be surprised, then, that cancer is not inherited directly, but as a constitution which allows cancer.

The connections between gene and tumor do not always have to be shrouded in mystery. Relatively simple analyses are possible in tumors which appear when closely related species are crossed.

Tumor Induction by Species Crossing: Tumor-Bearing Hybrids

In the animal and plant kingdoms there are numerous examples of tumor formation from special species crosses. Species crossing in cabbage *(Brassica)* causes a disposition toward tumors which are then induced by soil bacteria. Tumor-bearing hybrids can also be induced in thorn apples, snapdragons, calanchoe, tomatoes, barley, and other plants. Best known is the "preparation" of plant tumors with tobacco hybrids. If *Nicotiana glauca* is crossed with *Nicotiana langsdorffii*, tumors develop in the F_1 hybrids, in the root and in the sprout (see page 234).

Tumor induction by hybridization in animals is no rarity either. They are known in crosses of ducks, chickens, mice, butterflies, and gray horses. The most extensive investigations have been on crosses between swordtail fishes. Here, most is known about the formation of melanomas (Gordon, Anders).

In the first generation, the cross between the swordtails *Platypoecilus maculatus* and *Xiphophorus helleri* (both from Central America) leads to an expansion in the black, melanin-containing spots on the dorsal fin. The reddish shimmering areas in the neighborhood of the black spots also get bigger (Figure 43).

If this hybrid is backcrossed with an unspotted *Xiphophorus*, new hybrids can be produced with extensive melanin spots soon after birth. In addition, almost the entire body of the fish is covered with a red color. Within a few weeks the spots turn into melanomas, which finally kill the fish (Figure 44).

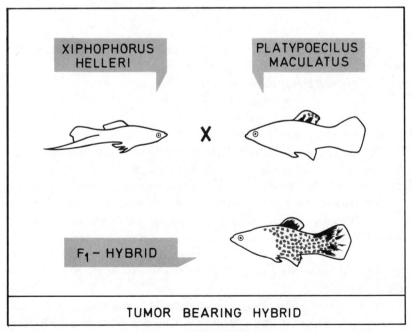

XIPHOPHORUS HELLERI

PLATYPOECILUS MACULATUS

X

F₁ – HYBRID

TUMOR BEARING HYBRID

Figure 43

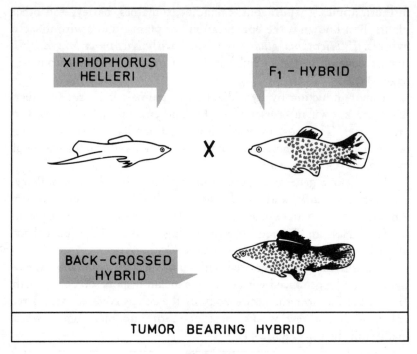

| XIPHOPHORUS HELLERI | F₁ – HYBRID |

| BACK–CROSSED HYBRID | |

TUMOR BEARING HYBRID

Figure 44

Although these melanomas arise exclusively *via* genetic manipulation, they are true tumors. Recall a few criteria:

1. They are *transplantable*.
2. They can grow *invasively*.
3. They *metastasize* in certain gene combinations.
4. They show aerobic glycolysis.

Obviously there is an unbalanced equilibrium here: neither parental genetic material is capable of holding the melanophores (pigment cells) of the hybrids under control. These are only crude qualitative considerations; closer genetic analysis reveals that an upset balance is not involved, but that regulating genes of one partner are increasingly diluted by breeding in nonregulating genes of the other partner.

Let us look first at a highly simplified gene analysis of the two partners. We need three genes to describe this case of genetic constitution (Figure 45):

1. A *pigment gene* (FG) is responsible for the formation of the macromelanophores in *Platypoecilus maculatus.* Naturally, this gene cannot by itself decide whether pigment cells are formed or not.

"Modification" genes, which decide whether the information of the pigment gene is actually put to use, are necessary. Two different gene systems come under consideration:

2. *Repressor genes* (RG) suppress the activity of the pigment gene or at least limit it greatly. This is the case with *P. maculatus*. It is known that these repressor genes are on a chromosome other than that of the pigment gene. We must therefore assume that the repressor regulated by these genes normally permits only a well-dosed action of the pigment gene.

3. In addition to these "braking genes" there are "acceleration genes" *(Inducer genes* = IG). These genes promote the turning out of melanophores, probably in a very unspecific manner. They increase the amino acid supply and also regulate the constitution of the amino acid pool.

Using these genes we can describe the genetic constitution of *Platypoecilus, Xiphophorus,* and their hybrids, and thus make the production of melanomas understandable (Figure 45).

We have continually talked about pigment genes. In fact, not only is the synthesis of melanin deregulated, but also the "synthesis" of the melanin-forming cells themselves, the melanophores. Thus we could speak of an error in regulation of cell division of these melanophores. The so-called pigment genes would accordingly be primarily growth genes instead. These growth genes are sufficiently repressed in the normal case; in the back-crossed hybrid this brake has escaped.

We can also describe this material using "chalone" terminology (see pp. 77 ff.): according to Bullough, chalones are tissue-specific substances produced in the tissue itself which suppress the growth rate of the tissue.

Using this chalone concept, models for a tumor cell can be proposed:

a) A cell can be under the influence of a meager supply of chalone. Cells under chalone deficiency conditions should divide faster than normal cells.

b) In some manner, direct or indirect, chalones must influence DNA synthesis and mitosis. Obviously the intervention of an acceptor is necessary. If this acceptor is damaged or completely inactivated, then the chalones cannot attack, and the tissue specific brake on mitosis doesn't function.

But let us get back to our fish hybrids and their genes: the repressor gene corresponds to the chalone producer and thus indirectly to

PLATYPOECILUS MACULATUS

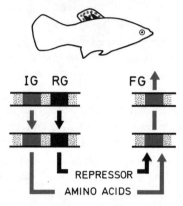

Pigment genes (PG) are inhibited by repressor gene (RG). Color production *via* unspecific induction (IG) cannot proceed over this inhibition.

XIPHOPHORUS HELLERI

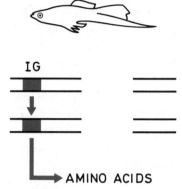

X. helleri has not developed a pigment gene during evolution, and hence also lacks a pigment repressor. Unspecific induction genes are present, however.

F₁ - HYBRID

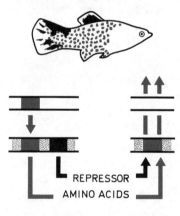

Partial derepression of pigment genes due to lack of repressor. The induction genes now effect an increase in spots and tumors.

BACK - CROSSED HYBRID

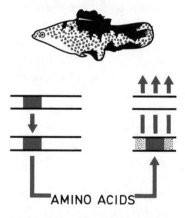

Major derepression of pigment genes, since repressor genes are now lacking completely. The influence of the induction genes leads here to rapidly growing melanomas (from Anders et al.)

Figure 45

the chalone. The pigment gene corresponds to the chalone acceptor. Loss of the repressor (chalone) can then lead directly to elevated division and development of the tumor.

Let us list once more the changes in genetic material which we have learned to this point:

1. Changes in the chromosome complement and the form of individual chromosomes are direct indications in many tumors of an altered genetic material (Philadelphia chromosome).

2. Breeding of tumorous strains depends on the preexistence of altered genes. In a large animal population, obviously enough immediately hidden gene mutants are present which lead finally to cancer and only have to be concentrated by breeding.

3. The breeding of hybrids also leads to alteration in the genetic material by substitution of related but not identical chromosomes or chromosome sections.

Until now we have excluded "artificial" carcinogenesis and must now ask again what role heredity plays in the induction of tumors by such things as irradiation or chemicals.

"Artificial" Carcinogenesis and Heredity

If methylcholanthrene is injected intramuscularly into mice, sarcomas develop. In a mixed mouse population there are animals which react strongly and others which get no tumors at all. If these extremes are selected out, strains can be bred with high and low sensitivity to methylcholanthrene respectively.

These and other experiments force us to conclude that artificial tumor induction is also dependent on the genetic constitution of the animal. Here, as with spontaneous tumors, "genetic constitution" can mean many things and among them the loss of the capability to activate carcinogen and incompetent or overcompetent immune system. In a hypothetical environment in which methylcholanthrene is always present at a constant level, genetic constitution alone would decide whether tumors appear or not. Thus the "hierarchy of causes" can be reversed: in a sensitive strain with a constant genetic constitution, the carcinogen is the "prime mover" of tumor induction; for animals under a constant dose level of carcinogen, it is heredity.

Occasionally carcinogen and inheritance appear to plow the same furrow: thus there are mice (0 28) with a genetically fixed lung cancer incidence (about 30 percent after 12 months). After "supplemental" treatment with diethylnitrosamine, 90 percent of the mice come down with bronchial carcinoma (Mohr).

Hence, genetic constitution guarantees a deciding contribution in the transformation of a normal cell into a tumor cell by a carcinogenic stimulus. But we can go one step further and ask if the carcinogens themselves do not react with the genetic material.

Consider once more the tumor-bearing swordtail hybrids in Figure 45. Here the repressors which control cell growth were "diluted out" or completely eliminated by crossing. The same effect ought to be realized if the production of the repressor were tied up by direct attack on the repressor gene. But such an attack is nothing other than a mutation.

This is the substance of the mutation theory of malignant growth (K. H. Bauer, 1928; Whitman, 1919): carcinogenic stimuli (irradiation, carcinogens) cause mutations; mutations in the growth-regulating portions of the genetic material are responsible for the neoplastic properties of a tumor cell. (Purists would rather refer to this as the mutation *hypothesis.*)

These carcinogen-induced mutations take place naturally in somatic cells and not in the germ cells. This means that the changes can be transmitted to the daughters of the mutated cell, but not to the offspring of the animal. The mutation theory of cancer is thus occasionally given the more exact name, theory of "somatic mutations."

Mutagenic and Carcinogenic Activity can be Correlated

Good mutagens should be good carcinogens, and *vice versa,* if the mutation theory is correct. It has long been known that X-rays are both carcinogenic and mutagenic; the same holds true for the softer ultra-violet rays. Not only radiation has this "dual identity"; a whole series of chemical mutagens are simultaneously carcinogens. A well-known example is mustard gas.

The correlation between mutagenicity and carcinogenicity is quite good in the nitrosamine series: the better the carcinogen, the more mutagenic it is. Of course this proof is somewhat less convincing when one considers that the carcinogenicity test is carried out on rats, while the mutagenicity is determined in *Drosophila.* These fundamentally incommensurable test systems are the real crux of any experimental test of the gene mutation hypothesis.

This criticism applies to most of the comprehensive listings in which the carcinogenic and mutagenic activities of various substances are compared. Thus it is not really surprising when occasionally substances are described which are mutagenic but not carcinogenic, or the reverse.

Methylcholanthrene is an excellent carcinogen in mice and other systems. The mutation rate, also in mice, is hardly increased, however. X-rays also show considerable quantitative differences: an irradiated animal reacts much more sensitively with mutations than with tumors — the exact reverse of the methylcholanthrene situation. A true apologist for the mutation theory has a convincing objection at hand here, too: somatic mutations are really something different from mutations in the germ cells. Only anatomic topography would validate such an assumption.

In the strictest sense, it would be permissible only to compare the carcinogenic effects of a substance with its ability to cause somatic mutations. Smith used tobacco for such a rigorous comparison: he induced tumors in certain tobacco hybrids with radiation. In the same plant, the irradiation simultaneously induces somatic mutations of certain pigmentation genes. Mutation and carcinogenesis each went its own way; they acted on different target cells. Now plant tumors do not find much favor in the eyes of many physicians. But in animals, too, (*Drosophila* again) the attempt to establish a direct relationship between somatic mutations and the appearance of tumors was a failuré.

Here, too, there are good counterarguments to keep the mutation theory from being shot down. Assume that some procedure or substance causes mutations in somatic cells, influencing production of pigments or bringing about some other "visible" change. Some, however, would transform a cell to a tumor cell ("growth regulation mutants"). This tumor cell would then have tremendous selective advantage over other somatic mutants: it produces cells of its own stamp in increasing measure. The other mutants would have to follow the normal division rhythm of the tissue, i. e., in the usual case they would multiply rarely. Hence it should be a rare event to come across a mutated somatic cell, while it should not be at all unusual to stumble upon a tumor cell. It is easy to forget that even a macroscopically visible tumor is derived from a microscopic base, just as invisible in the beginning as many of the somatic mutations.

Hence, clear correlations ought always to be exceptions.

Mutation Hypothesis as a Theoretical Necessity

The gene mutation hypothesis is still waiting for unequivocal experimental proof. This does not mean that this theory has been pigeonholed, however. On the contrary, it is as vital as ever, simply because it is almost a theoretical necessity:

1. Tumor cells transmit their neoplastic properties to their daughter cells. Thus the genetic material of the cell appears to be responsible in the final analysis.

2. In the overwhelming majority of cases, the conversion of a normal cell into a cancer cell is irreversible. The route to cancer is a road of no return.

Both criteria, "genetic memory" and irreversibility, also hold for classic mutation. Other "genetic mechanisms" such as permanent modifications consequently appear to be excluded (but see Pitot and Heidelberger, *Cancer Research*, 1963). However, at this point we have reached a form of circular definition: mutations have the same properties as neoplastic change. Whether all carcinogens are really mutagens now appears to be a question of secondary importance, particularly since there are thoroughly convincing arguments to explain why the correlation between mutagenesis and carcinogenesis must always have exceptions.

Objections to the Mutation Theory

For a long time virus tumors were a favorite argument against the mutation theory. It is thought that they do not permit an explanation of their genesis on the basis of a gene mutation. Lately these tumors are in fact being used to support the mutation theory. Naturally mutation in this context is not meant in the sense of an alteration of the already present genetic material, but it is surely not incorrect to speak of mutations, of a change in the genetic material, when a virus genome has incorporated into the cell genome. And of course there are not only point mutations in classical genetics either. This new-found love between mutation theory and virology was not awakened at all by new experiments or surprising findings. The "novel" facts have been known and discussed for a long time. But old feuds can simply be laid to rest.

A second objection to the mutation theory is also losing more and more substance: tumor induction is a slow, occasionally extremely slow process. Manifestation of a *mutation,* however, is a rapid, even *very rapid process.*

Perhaps the two-step experiment (pp. 53 ff.) will facilitate understanding of this apparent paradox. Recall that it is possible to induce "latent" tumor cells by a single (subthreshold) application of a carcinogen, and that these latent tumor cells can be "developed" into a true tumor with a non-carcinogenic tumor promotor. It would then be conceivable that the first rapid induction of latent tumor cells (initiation) has something to do with a mutative process, whereas tumor promotion proceeds without mutations.

Simply the fact that DAB has to be fed for an extended period, to get hepatomas, gave rise to the suspicion that one "hit" — carcinogen against genetic material — does not do the job. Close quantitative analyses showed that we must reckon with many hits. We can thus speak of a carcinogenesis as a *multiple-hit reaction.* The latent period would then simply be the time required for a sufficient number of hits.

Concluding Words on the Mutation Theory

"The insight that a cancer cell is a mutated cell belongs without doubt to the fundamental advances in the area of tumor research" (Euler). "It has today become commonplace to say that a hereditary change is involved in the conversion of a normal cell to a tumor cell" (Schultz). Both quotations come from "Das Krebsproblem," a book by K. H. Bauer which, in his words, "is dictated by the spirit and language of the mutation theory."

But let us hear some more quotations: "We have to recognize that the question of whether cancer can be considered a mutation is not answered. If all scientifically established facts are viewed, which argue for or against the mutation theory, it must be admitted that the balance is tipped in favor of the latter side" (Heston). Oberling cites this statement in his "Rätsel des Krebses." It is Oberling's opinion that "cancer is naturally a mutation, if one considers every cell alteration which is heritable a mutation". He goes on: "If we do not want to be deluded by the 'word,' 'which shows up just in time,' we must try to define the mutation concept more sharply." Then, against the background of a mutation theory which he believes to have foundered, Oberling develops with that much more energy the general virus theory.

Objectively, the problem remains undecided. Any decisions are strongly colored by prejudices, but even a strong dose of prejudice has never hurt a good working hypothesis. A single classical mutation is probably not enough for production of a tumor cell. But just as surely it appears that the decisive changes must be played out in the genetic material, which means that carcinogens must react with cellular DNA. Thus, some aspects of the interactions of carcinogens with DNA will be presented in the next chapter.

Summary

There are good reasons for assuming that the decisive changes in the conversion of a normal cell to a tumor cell are alterations in the genetic material.

1. These changes are immediately visible in deviated chromosome patterns (Boveri's chromosome theory of malignant tumors). Occasionally certain neoplasms are distinguished by a characteristically altered chromosome; a well-known example is the Philadelphia chromosome in chronic myeloid leukemia. Tumors with normal chromosome complements make generalization difficult, however.

2. Altered genetic material that leads to tumors as a final consequence can be isolated by breeding. The animal strains thus obtained, with 100 percent incidence of a given spontaneous tumors, are an important tool in experimental oncology. They clearly show that cancer is heritable, although there has been no success in finding simple genetic connections between tumor frequency and tumor type. Cancer as such is not inherited — only a provision for it, but this is a commonplace in genetics.

3. Occasionally simple species crosses lead to tumors. Examples of tumor-bearing hybrids are found in both botany and zoology. Genetic analysis shows that regulator genes in one of the species may be more or less diluted out by crossing.

4. The mutation theory of cancer (Bauer, 1928) postulates that carcinogenic stimuli, whether of chemical or physical nature, lead to mutations in somatic cells. These mutations must involve growth-regulating functions. This is the simplest interpretation of the "genetic memory" of a cell, which ensures that cancer cells of the same type arise from a parent cancer cell. Experimental proof of this theoretically almost necessary concept is still to be desired.

DNA AND CARCINOGENESIS

Life hangs by a thread, in an entirely literal sense. Monstrously long DNA chains regulate structure and function of a bacteria as well as in mammalian cells. (The DNA fibers of a single mouse cell, if strung out in one thread would be almost a meter long.) For the chemist they are really quite simple fibers (polynucleotides); polyester fibers, the plastics chemist would call them, hardly more complicated than Nylon or Dacron.

But DNA molecules are very "special" fibers: their four building blocks are only seemingly in random order; they code the approximately 20 amino acids of the proteins (genetic code), with three nucleotides equivalent to a given amino acid (triplet code). In reading off this molecular Morse code, the information of tle DNA tape is first played onto an RNA tape (messenger RNA; transcription). The transcribing enzymes are RNA polymerases. Deciphering then takes place at the ribosomes: here the individual amino acids are towed to the correct places on the messenger RNA by porters (transfer RNA; translation).

All of these processes are quite complex, but their end result is basically simple: amino acids are fed as a mixture into a black box which they leave coupled together in a definite order. DNA dictates style in this box. The amino acid sequences are unequivocally defined by the nucleotide sequences of the DNA (the "central dogma" of molecular biology).

DNA does more for a cell than determine protein sequences. DNA can cause identical copies of itself to be produced (principle of complementary double strands), and consequently as genetic material guarantee the identical replication of a cell.

The two processes, replication of DNA and direction of protein synthesis, are closely related. In both cases a new strand is complementarily constructed on an unwound DNA double strand. If this new strand consists of deoxyribonucleotides, then an identical copy of the original double strand comes out. If ribonucleotides are polymerized, then messenger RNA (or ribosomal RNA) molecules result, which in their turn undertake protein synthesis.

In experimental cancer research, the DNA became of interest primarily as genetic material, for if tumor cells are viewed as a new strain of cells, then it must also be assumed that tumor cells have "new" genetic material at their disposal.

Tumor DNA as a Carcinogen

It ought to be possible to produce tumor cells using a simple recipe: treat normal cells with a DNA preparation from tumor cells and transmit directly the "new" genetic material into normal cells. Cantarow has done such experiments: he prepared DNA from hepatomas, incubated cells from regenerating liver with this preparation, and then injected the treated liver cells directly into livers of rats. After about 12 weeks he found tumors at the site of injection, although in very low yield.

As yet, however, such reports remain exceptional: the neoplastic transformation of normal cells with tumor DNA has not yet been brought off more generally. The nucleic acid preparations usually have only a cytotoxic effect: quantities of nucleic acid greater than 200 µg/ml are lethal for the cells of a cell culture. Why does transformation by tumor DNA cause such difficulties? In bacteria the transmission of genetic properties with DNA preparations has become routine procedure since Avery.

The cells of higher organisms seem to behave differently from bacteria. In 1956 the apparently unbelievable report was spread that ducks had been genetically altered with DNA injections. In Strasbourg DNA from the Khaki Campbell breed of ducks had been isolated and injected into white pekingeses. The offspring of the pekingeses, it was said, showed a few peculiarities of the Campbell ducks. Later the Strasbourg duck story proved to be for the birds, but successful experiments on *Drosophila* and on cells in tissue culture have since been reported.

The transformation of higher cells with DNA is obviously a ticklish matter — but why, really? It is not that DNA is not taken up into the cells, for it has been successfully demonstrated that DNA can move into the cells as a macromolecule. To be sure, most of it (80 percent) gets hung up on the cell surface; only a very small portion actually enters the cell interior. The cell itself does not appear to give any enzymatic help: even at 0 °C DNA is still taken up.

Naturally there are definite differences between a bacterial cell and a mammalian cell, especially in construction of the genetic substance: simple DNA fibers in the case of bacteria, complicated chromosomal structures in higher cells. It ought to be obvious that it is a problem for a DNA fiber to insinuate itself into a chromosome. There is an important exception to this "rule," however.

Infectious Tumor Virus DNA, a Potent "Chemical Carcinogen"

Infectious DNA can be isolated from polyoma virus, meaning that cells can be infected as well with this DNA as with intact virus. The usual plaques arise in cell layers, which can be counted. These DNA preparations are also carcinogenic: if they are injected into newborn hamsters, tumors develop.

Why can virus DNA do that which comes so hard to tumor DNA? It would be conceivable that the virus DNA "knows" how to fit into the host genome, while normal DNA is simply sensed as a macromolecular foreign body to be gotten rid of.

It is very probable that the decision is made on the way to the cell: the serum of a mouse inactivates bacterial DNA within a few minutes, while polyoma DNA remains untouched. Consequently polyoma DNA has a good chance of hitting a sensitive cell and transforming it.

From the standpoint of the chemist, this DNA is a "chemical carcinogen" in the strictest sense. Its building blocks are exactly defined, the mode of connection is known, and it is known how many have been assembled in a polydeoxyribonucleotide. Of course the many easily cleaved ester bonds between the individual deoxynucleotides make this carcinogen highly vulnerable, and its considerable size makes entrance into a cell difficult.

Still, polyoma DNA has a definite advantage over the classical carcinogens such as 3,4-benzpyrene: it obviously contains all the information necessary to "redirect" a normal cell. Like a treacherous pilot, it steers the ship aground intentionally. Benzpyrene and the other chemical carcinogens first have to get a hand on the regulation hierarchy of the cell, meaning they have to get to the DNA.

Carcinogens Disturb DNA Synthesis

After application of carcinogenic substances, it is often observed that DNA synthesis falls. If carcinogenic hydrocarbons are painted on the back of a mouse or fed to a mouse, a short-term inhibition of DNA synthesis in the skin is observed in both cases. After the depression there follows a period of increased new DNA synthesis.

There is a general tendency not to attach too much significance to either effect in carcinogenesis. They are simply chalked up as "toxic side effects," and it is thought that an injury is followed by regeneration of the damaged cells. But carcinogens do not simply cause trouble in DNA synthesis.

Carcinogens Disturb the Formation of Adaptive Enzymes

Adaptive enzymes are enzymes produced only when a cell needs them. Many examples are known, especially in microorganisms, but a liver, too, produces certain enzymes only on demand: thus tryptophane induces the tryptophane-catabolizing enzyme tryptophane pyrrolase, tyrosine induces tyrosine transaminase, etc. (substrate induction). Carcinogens can inhibit this induction: DAB and acetylaminofluorene hinder the induction of tryptophane pyrrolase by tryptophane (Pitot).

Carcinogens can also interfere with more complicated induction processes: glucose-6-phosphatase is induced by cortisone in the liver, and this hormonal induction is also blocked, by the carcinogenic 3'-methyl-DAB. If we assume, in analogy to the regulatory processes in bacteria, that in the induction of enzymes, previously suppressed DNA information is transcribed, this conclusion follows: carcinogens disorder the transcription of DNA.

A similar result was obtained by de Maeyer in a completely different system. Investigating the influence of carcinogenic and noncarcinogenic hydrocarbons on virus production in cell cultures, he found that carcinogenic substances can inhibit the production of DNA viruses, but not of RNA viruses. Noncarcinogenic hydrocarbons were without effect in either case. These findings also suggest that the transcription of DNA can be disordered by carcinogens.

A blockade of DNA information would mean that the synthesis of messenger RNA was limited or even completely shut off. Biochemically speaking, this means that the DNA dependent RNA polymerases have difficulties with carcinogen-modified DNA.

RNA polymerases can be obtained pure. Using such pure enzymes, one can conduct RNA synthesis from DNA in a test tube. Only pure enzyme, RNA building blocks (adenosine triphosphate, guanosine triphosphate, etc.), and a DNA template are required. The DNA is important, for without it the RNA polymerase cannot assemble the building blocks into an RNA chain.

Troll has compared DNA from normal liver with DNA from "carcinogen-treated" liver, and found that the "carcinogen DNA" was less well suited to "prime" RNA synthesis than was normal DNA. Thus it was shown that carcinogens can in fact make transcription of DNA information more difficult.

A simple explanation would be that carcinogens are bound directly to the DNA and there like barbs interrupt the sliding past of the RNA polymerase.

Chemical Carcinogens React with the Cell DNA

For a long time this reaction had been overlooked. For years interest was focused almost exclusively on the binding of chemical carcinogens to soluble proteins, and a key reaction in the conversion of a normal cell to a tumor cell was seen in this coupling. Even today this idea is still very much prevalent, but through the years people have become uncertain. More and more observations failed to fit these concepts.

1. Baldwin reported that the heterocyclic carcinogen tricycloquinazoline is hardly bound at all to soluble protein, and of that is primarily bound to albumin and not to h-protein.

2. The binding of carcinogens to soluble proteins can be reduced without reducing the tumor yield. Experiments of this type also suggest that protein-carcinogen complexes have no direct significance in carcinogenesis.

More and more, people began looking for reactions with DNA. In these researches it turned out that carcinogens were very probably able to react with cellular DNA. The more active the carcinogen, the more it was bound. Brookes studied the binding of carcinogenic and noncarcinogenic polycyclic hydrocarbons to DNA in mouse skin, and found that this binding closely followed the Iball indices (p. 44) for carcinogenic activity: naphthalene, with an index = 0 was not bound; 7,12-dimethylbenzanthracene, with the highest index in the series, was bound the best (1 molecule per 25,000 nucleotides).

An observation by Colburn and Boutwell also supports the hypothesis that the binding of carcinogens to DNA has something to do with carcinogenesis. They found that β-propiolactone, an initiator for skin tumors, at differing doses induces tumors in direct proportion to its binding to mouse skin DNA.

The form in which polycyclic hydrocarbons are bound is not yet known; the situation is better for other carcinogens.

Covalent Bonds between Carcinogens and Guanine

The preferred binding partner among the building blocks of DNA is guanine, one of the purine bases. Let us look at a few examples:

Mustard gas reacts with the "upper" nitrogen in the 5-membered ring (N_7):

This reaction follows the general rules of alkylation (see p. 203). β-Propiolactone is similarly bound to guanine:

Acetylaminofluorene is also bound to guanine, but on the 8-carbon atom:

Methylnitrosourea again alkylates the N_7 of guanine:

Reactions other than these are known to take place (alkylation of adenine, binding to the 6-oxygen of guanine), and there is some speculation that these reactions, rather than the predominant reactions mentioned, may be the critical reactions leading to carcinogenesis.

Eventual Consequences of the Reactions with Guanine

Even the small alteration in guanine (G) resulting from introduction of a methyl group can have far-reaching consequences for the DNA. Nitrogen-1 becomes more acid, i. e., the bond between this atom and its hydrogen atom becomes weaker. Instead of the normal base-pairing G—C, the wrong pairing G(methyl)-T can take place.

$$G — C \longrightarrow \boxed{G} — T$$

At first this is only a small error, but it is retained in all future DNA generations, for during the next replication, an A is introduced instead of the original G into the complementary strand:

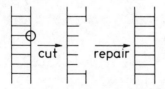

As the final result, then, a G—C pair would be replaced by an A—T pair. A mistake would have crept into both strands (mutation). Of course, the DNA has not been left completely helpless against such damage.

Cells can Repair Defective DNA

Bacterial geneticists had discovered that radiation damaged DNA can be put in order again by the cell. We now know that such repairs can also be carried out in mammalian cells:

If cells are given radioactive thymidine (one of the four building blocks of DNA) during such a repair process, it is built into the repaired DNA sections and can easily be demonstrated. An apparent new synthesis takes place, although in reality pieces of DNA are only being mended. (This apparent new synthesis can naturally be carried out independently of the S-phase of the cell cycle, and is therefore occasionally referred to as "unscheduled DNA synthesis.")

It is suggestive to assume that these mending mechanisms also play a role in carcinogenesis: cells without a repair system or with a poor one ought to be especially susceptible to carcinogenic effects. Such cells have in fact been discovered: fibroblasts isolated from the skin of patients with the genetic disease *Xeroderma pigmentosum* showed a defective repair system. Hence, light-caused damage suffered by the genomes of these cells cannot be corrected. Cells from *Xeroderma pigmentosum* patients are not the only example of a possible connection between "repairases" and tumor induction. Repair enzymes also appear to play an important role in the so-called carcinogenesis in vitro.

Neoplastic Transformations Work Better with Proliferating Cells

Normal cells of a culture in vitro can be converted to tumor cells with carcinogenic stimuli such as chemical carcinogens, irradiation, and with tumor viruses. There is one important limitation on this transformation in vitro: it hardly goes, if at all, when one attempts

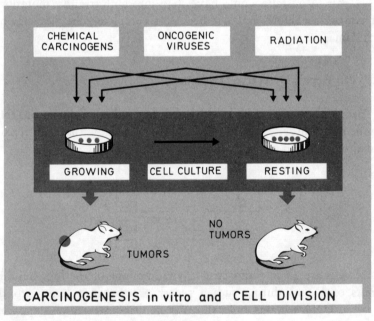

Figure 46

to transform resting cells which have reached confluent density. But if a cell culture is treated which has not reached this stage and whose cells are still dividing, then transformation succeeds. The same cell culture is sensitive when "young" and proliferating, but insensitive when "old" and resting (Sachs) (see Figure 46).

Observations of this kind have been made not only on in vitro transformation:

1. The induction of leukemias by X-rays works most easily when the target cells (bone marrow cells, for example) are most intensively dividing. This is the case during embryonic development, and it is thus evident that fetuses have an especially high risk.

2. An example of a plant tumor (crown gall) also reveals that the transformation of a cell into a tumor cell has something to do with its "proliferation status." Crown gall can be induced by infecting plants with a certain bacterium *(B. tumefaciens).*

However, the mere presence of the bacterium will not transform normal cells unless the plant has been conditioned — that is, made suspectible — by means of a wound inflicted on its tissues. In other words, the principle takes effect only if the cells have been subjected to the irritation accompanying a wound. Moreover, the effect is not a one-step process. Cells transformed about 34 hours after the wound has been inflicted are benign and grow only slowly. If the transformation takes place about 50 hours after the wound, the tumor cells grow somewhat faster. In contrast, cells that are transformed between 60 and 72 hours after wounding grow very rapidly and are fully autonomous. Detailed examination has disclosed that this drastic transformation occurs if the change is induced at the stage in the wound-healing cycle just before the normal plant cells begin to divide most actively in the process of repairing the wound (A. Braun).

Reparases could be the reason why resting cells are so much less sensitive: in resting cells the reparases have time to cut out the mistakes in the DNA caused by the carcinogens, and replace them by a mistake-free strand. Thus the effect of the carcinogen is lost. In contrast, in cells in which the DNA synthesis phases follow closely upon each other, an error can be transmitted to the newly synthesized strand, "fixing" the carcinogenic effect (see above).

Thus this would explain why only cells which duplicate their DNA soon after contact with a carcinogenic stimulus have a chance of being transformed. The gradations in malignancy of plant tumor cells can also be explained by assuming that the attack of a carcinogen on a highly proliferating tissue can introduce more permanent hits. In these tumors it is very probably not the bacterium, but an accompanying virus which is the actual carcinogen, but this does not alter the point of these considerations.

Binding without Bonds: Intercalation

The best-known example for such noncovalent, loose attachments are the acridine orange dyes. These dye molecules wedge themselves between the bases of the DNA double helix as flat discs. This results in false base-pairing during replication and consequently in mutations.

The classical carcinogens, especially the polycyclic hydrocarbons, can also *intercalate*. In in vitro experiments primarily, it could be shown that the hydrocarbons can be squeezed into DNA molecules. Pyrene works best in such a system, but unfortunately pyrene is noncarcinogenic. Thus it is doubtful that intercalation by itself has a very large role in carcinogenesis.

Summary

The "new properties" of a tumor cell should be tied to the genetic material (DNA) of the cell. The simple transfer of tumor properties with tumor DNA is a controversial matter, however; tumor DNA is a carcinogen of highly questionable reputation. DNA from tumor viruses is a recognized carcinogen, however.

The binding of carcinogens to DNA might play an important role in chemical carcinogenesis:

1. Better carcinogens are bound better to DNA.
2. The degree of binding (at least in the case of β-propiolactone) is correlated with tumor yield. But these experiments, too, are indications at best.

In a few cases, the exact mode of binding between carcinogen and DNA is known. The preferred binding partner is guanine, especially through alkylation at N_7.

In isolated cases, intercalation could play a role.

The transformation of a normal cell into a tumor cell depends on the "proliferation status" of the affected cell: cells in division are converted to tumor cells more easily than are resting cells. A possible explanation was discussed: repair enzymes have sufficient time in resting cells to mend the injury caused by the carcinogenic stimulus, before the alteration can be "fixed" by the next DNA replication.

A FEW MODELS FOR TUMOR CHEMOTHERAPY

The recipes for success from chemotherapy of bacterial disease cannot be applied to the battle against tumor cells: the penicillins, for example, block the synthesis of the bacterial cell wall without disturbing the cell membranes of a mammalian cell. But in spite of all their differences, the tumor cell and the normal cell are both mammalian cells. Thus there was pessimism everywhere concerning the possibility of finding substances which would selectively kill tumor cells. But in 1946, success was reported: Hodgkin's disease had been successfully treated with nitrogen mustard. Nitrogen mustard is a highly toxic compound, though, and extreme care in dosage was required. Still, people began to prepare compounds of similar types, and it was hoped that substances could soon be found that could kill tumor cells without causing too great damage to the normal cells of a normal tissue. By now, over a quarter of a million chemical compounds have been synthesized and tested for effectiveness against tumors, not one of which was a "wonder drug." In spite of this, many of these chemotherapeutic agents have their merits; a few of them have secured a place alongside the surgeon's knife and the radiologist's high energy beams.

The more we know about the fine line between tumor cells and normal cells, the easier it will be to find tailor-made chemotherapeutic agents. For a long time, the elevated rate of division of tumor cells has been considered the most conspicuous characteristic and most susceptible aspect. The best-known of our chemotherapeutic agents are therefore substances that attack DNA synthesis.

Alkylating Agents

A chemistry student learns the meaning of alkylation practically the first day he walks into organic chemistry lab. He mixes methyl iodide with ethanol and gets ethyl methyl ether.

In another example he produces mono-, di-, and triethylamine from ethyl iodide and ammonia:

$$C_2H_5I + NH_3 \rightarrow H_2NC_2H_5 \text{ etc.}$$

In both examples a hydrogen atom is replaced by an alkyl residue (methyl or ethyl). CH_3I and C_2H_5I are alkylating agents; ethanol and ammonia have been alkylated.

Alkylating substances play a large role in the tool chest of the synthetic chemist. Their reactivity makes them indispensable aids in the synthesis of many compounds. In fact, they really belong in the poison cabinet: they react aggressively with cell components and block vital cell functions. In World War I, some especially reactive alkylating agents were used as chemical weapons, especially mustard gas:

$$S\diagup\diagdown\begin{matrix}CH_2CH_2Cl\\CH_2CH_2Cl\end{matrix}$$

Besides severe burning of the skin and fatal lung damage (due to the hydrochloric acid liberated), even then severe damage was noticed primarily in rapidly proliferating tissues, such as the intestinal mucosa and the bone marrow. In World War II, there was also an opportunity to study the effect on blood cells. A supply ship loaded with 100 tons of mustard gas had tied up in the port of Bari, Italy. In an ensuing bombing attack, the ship was hit, releasing large quantities of the poison. People who suffered contact died immediately or later showed severe changes in the blood with a reduced leucocyte count (leucopenia).

Why shouldn't mustard gases also be able to effect a reduction in the lymphocyte excess associated with leukemia? The classical sulfur mustard was too toxic for therapeutic purposes, but a compound varying only slightly, the so-called nitrogen mustard

$$CH_3 - N\diagup\diagdown\begin{matrix}CH_2CH_2Cl\\CH_2CH_2Cl\end{matrix}$$

has demonstrated its worth against a few forms of leukemic diseases. It has not since gained any greater significance.

Nitrogen Mustard with a Fuse

The highly reactive mustard compounds have difficulty in reaching the tumor; while under way they react with other cells and serum components. To get around this difficulty, people searched for derivatives that would release active mustard only to the tumor (principle of latent activity). The best-known compound of this type is cyclophosphamide (Endoxan),

$$
\begin{array}{c}
CH_2-NH \\
CH_2 \qquad\qquad P-N \\
CH_2-O
\end{array}
\begin{array}{c}
O \\
\| \\
\end{array}
\begin{array}{c}
CH_2CH_2Cl \\
CH_2CH_2Cl
\end{array}
$$

in which the nitrogen is made part of a cyclic phosphamide ester (Arnold). It was hoped that the phosphate ester would preferentially be taken up by the rapidly proliferating tumor cells and only there be activated. In fact, however, Endoxan is activated in the liver. Direct attack on tumor cells was hardly ever seen. The hope of finding a relatively nontoxic, tumor-specific mustard compound, remained unfulfilled. Still, Endoxan is one of the materials most effective against a broad spectrum of experimental tumors.

Direct Attack on Tumor DNA

Alkylating agents react with all "alkylatable" compounds; they react with proteins and with nucleic acids. People today are inclined to believe that the reaction with DNA is the key reaction for the biological effect. Guanine and adenine are alkylated, chain breakage follows and even cross-linking (in the case of the bidentate mustards). It is obvious that a severely damaged DNA can no longer be replicated.

Alkylating agents represent a heavy-handed approach. There is, however, an indirect method of arriving at an effective inhibition of DNA synthesis.

Antimetabolites in Tumor Therapy

Metabolites of all sorts are produced in cell metabolism: protein intermediates (amino acids), nucleic acid building blocks (nucleotides), etc. Chemists have prepared a whole series of slightly altered metabolites that closely resemble the true metabolites, differing only in one or more small details. A well-known example of such an antimetabolite is 6-mercaptopurine (6 MP) (Hitchings),

$$SH \qquad\qquad NH_2$$

6 MP   Adenine

which resembles adenine in almost every respect. If such a false nucleic acid building block — like a Trojan horse — were to be incorporated into DNA, there would have to be some effect on DNA synthesis.

6-Mercaptopurine is in fact incorporated into RNA and DNA, but its principle effect appears to be indirect. It is converted to the riboside phosphate (corresponding to a nucleotide) and as such inhibits the conversion of inosinic acid to adenylic acid,

Inosinic acid   Adenylic acid

a conversion necessary for nucleic acid synthesis. The enzyme responsible for this reaction is fooled by the 6 MP nucleotide, binding it, and thus cannot work on the correct substrate (inosinic acid). In addition, 6 MP blocks early steps in de novo purine synthesis, by giving a false message to the enzymes at these stages that there are enough purines present in the cell (false negative feedback of biosynthesis).

New synthesis of DNA is just as strongly hindered by these indirect effects. Thus tumor cells that have just been ordered to go into DNA synthesis are inhibited by 6 MP.

There is still another reason that mercaptopurine is a good tumor inhibitor: normal mammalian cells can easily catabolize 6 MP, converting it into 6-thiouric acid (using xanthine oxidases). In general, however, tumor cells have less xanthine oxidase and are thus exposed to the effect of 6 MP longer than are normal cells. In other words, 6 MP has a selective effect on tumor cells.

A whole series of other antimetabolites has been introduced to tumor therapy. Methotrexate (Farber) and fluorouracil (Heidelberger) are probably the best known and most effective:

Folic acid (Methotrexate)   (Fluoro) uracil

Methotrexate is an antagonist of folic acid (required for nucleotide synthesis); fluorouracil primarily interferes with methylation of uridine monophosphate to thymidine monophosphate, similarly an important step in DNA synthesis. Recently cytosine arabinoside has been used in tumor therapy: in this compound, ribose is replaced by arabinose.

Immunosuppressive Side Effects

All chemotherapeutic agents that we have become acquainted with so far, antimetabolites and alkylating substances, are toxic substances that also involve normal cells. Consequently there are narrow limits on dosage. Even more unpleasant than the side effects on normal cells is the effect of these substances on the immune system (an immunosuppressive effect): alkylating agents and antimetabolites reduce the ability of the immune system to handle foreign material. By the same token, they also reduce the possibility that this system can trap tumor cells. Thus therapy with cytotoxic substances is always a calculated risk: the tumor cells ought to be completely wiped out; no residue can be allowed to remain that the immune defenses have to clean up. Hence the search for nontoxic tumor inhibitors is a most urgent assignment. The first indication of success was obtained with a medication derived from *E. coli:* asparaginase.

Asparaginase Starves Tumor Cells

In 1953 Kidd made a surprising discovery: he had injected guinea pig serum into mice with experimental lymphomas and observed that the tumors regressed. Broome seized upon this observation and fractionated the guinea pig serum to see which fraction was responsible for this antitumor effect. He established that all of the active fractions contained the enzyme asparaginase, an enzyme which cleaves the amino acid asparagine into ammonia and aspartic acid.

But why was it the lymphoma cells that reacted to the asparaginase? The explanation was simple: these tumor cells require an external source of asparagine; they cannot produce it themselves. Therefore, asparaginase cuts them off from the vitally necessary supply of asparagine. Normal cells usually can produce their own asparagine, so that asparagine is not an "essential" amino acid for normal cells.

Guinea pig serum contains very little asparaginase (100,000 liters of serum would be necessary to treat one patient); horse serum has even less. However, fairly large quantities of asparaginase can be isolated from E. coli (Mashburn). Large-scale investigations have been undertaken with this bacterial enzyme, but there have not yet been any sensational results. Still, a new principle was introduced to chemotherapy: instead of the unspecific effect of cytotoxic substances, the directed starvation of a tumor cell. A harmless defect in a tumor cell, namely its inability to synthesize its own asparagine, is made fatal.

Labilization of Tumor Cells by Excessive Acid

Glycolyzing tumors produce lactic acid and thus shift the pH of their environment to the acid side and damaging themselves in the bargain. In the usual situation this acid excess is not very pronounced. It can be increased by a trick however: four grams glucose per kilogram are intravenously infused into a mouse over 100 minutes. In this way the glucose throughput through the glycolytic chain is increased greatly, resulting in a multiplied lactic acid production. Intratumoral pH measurements showed that pH values down as far as 5.8 can be reached. Killing of the tumor cells does not succeed however.

Many Tumor Cells are Especially Heat-sensitive

If tumor cells (Morris hepatoma 5121 or the Novikoff hepatoma) are heated to 43° C, their respiration as determined by oxygen consumption is reduced by two-thirds. Normal cells (regenerating liver in this model system) remain unaffected. DNA synthesis in overheated tumor cells is reduced even more dramatically: after two hours of preincubation, the incorporation of thymidine is reduced to 10 percent of the normal value. Here, too, normal cells (regenerating liver) proved to be insensitive.

Neither heat treatment alone nor artificial creation of an acid environment can cause tumors to regress, but if tumor cells are damaged by these "harmless attacks," very small doses of effective chemotherapeutic agents can effect complete killing of tumor cells.

Multistep Therapy

Those most occupied with the combination of the cancerolytic effects of overheating and overacidification have been von Ardenne and his collective. In one example, tumor cells were incubated in a nitrogen mustard-N-oxide solution $(3 \times 10^{-4} M)$ at pH 7.3 and $36°$ C (normal conditions) or at pH 6.3 and $40°$ C (labilizing conditions). If the number of killed cells (those cells which took up Trypan blue) were counted at varying time intervals, there was found to be a damatic difference between "normal" and "labilized" tumor cells. The two-pronged attack of "overacidification + hyperthermia" had increased the effect of the cytostatic agent 10-fold.

In the organism, normal cells (this is the important point) would be largely unaffected because:

1. A glucose shock does not cause acidification of normal tissue.

2. Normal cells are less heat sensitive. Of course the whole organism is quite heat sensitive: circulatory disorders seem almost unavoidable, and this naturally is a severe limitation to general application of the method.

Chain Reactions Lead to a "Natural" Cell Death

The lysosomes may possibly play a key role in multistep therapy. We have already encountered these "suicide packages" with their load of hydrolytic enzymes. The pH optimum of activity for these enzymes is well into the acid range (pH 5), so that they are largely ineffective at the pH value of normal tissue. If the lysosomes in a cell are damaged as a result of therapeutic treatment (von Ardenne infers), then the enzyme activation in a highly overacidified tumor tissue is so extensive that it makes a considerable contribution to damaging neighboring cells. Thus an injured cell will help to destroy its neighbors, these their neighbors, and so on. Once the destruction has been ignited, it spreads through the entire tumor tissue as a chain reaction. When the chain reaches the normal tissue, however, it is broken, since the normal tissue is not acid and the lysosomal enzymes cannot be activated.

This scheme naturally assumes glycolyzing tumors, and we have seen that all tumors do not have to show a marked degree of glycolysis. Disregarding these, however, a large number of tumors would still be susceptible to such an attack. It would then be a "natural method," because a similar mechanism (overheating and release of lysosomal enzymes) takes place in inflammation, with a similar melting away of damaged tissue. In tumor therapy it would then simply be a matter of "kindling" the physiological "trash fire." In von Ardenne's words: "The basic principle and goal of multistep therapy of cancer is to set off the natural cytolytic mechanisms, but strictly localized in the cancer tissue."

Virus Tumor Therapy?

"Virus remedies" really ought to help against viral tumors, but there is not too much one can do against viruses. Antibodies naturally help against viruses, as against microbial invasions. Killed or weakened virus can immunize, as in the oral polio vaccine, and protective immunizations are possible against leukemia viruses (see page 149).

A mammalian organism does have a second antivirus weapon in its arsenal: *interferon*. This is a protein produced by cells when they are attacked by a virus and which blocks virus replication. Unfortunately, interferon is species specific (mouse cells protected only by mouse interferon, rat cells by rat interferon, etc.). Thus we would need human interferon to do anything against influenza or the sniffles.

There is an elegant method for producing interferon indirectly: poly I/C (polyinosinic-polycytidylic acid) stimulates interferon production even without a virus. This artificial double-stranded RNA does not only interfere with virus production in cell culture, it has already proved itself in field tests against viral diseases.

Poly I/C has more merits than simply blocking virus production; it inhibits tumors, even those which were not assumed (at least as yet) to be virus-induced. Possibly the tumor-inhibitory effect has nothing to do with its antiviral effect: poly I/C unspecifically stimulates the immune defense system and thus the defense against tumor cells. This, too, permits an understanding of how tumor regressions can be brought about.

It should be noted that theoretically any treatment proved valuable against virus reproduction (such as the new drug amantadine), should not be expected to have any effect on a viral genome once it is incorporated into the host genome. Since this appears to be the critical step in induction of tumors by viruses, however, it is clear that although any of the above methods may be preventive, there should not be any reason that they could act on a tumor already present (with the exception of the immunostimulation induced by poly I/C).

The same holds true for the proposition that tumors induced by RNA viruses can be treated by inhibitors (Rifampicin derivatives) of RNA dependent DNA polymerase (see p. 177). This enzyme appears to be necessary for incorporation of the viral information into the host genome, but this process has long since taken place when the tumor is diagnosed. Hence, treatment with an inhibitor of RNA dependent DNA polymerase is like locking the barn door after the horse has been stolen. We hope this is not the case, but too much hope should not be held out for the success of this treatment.

A New Star?

In the middle of the twentieth century, surprised biologists made use of theological vocabulary and spoke of a "God of the amoebae" (Arndt). The basis of their fascination were observations they had made on cells of the slime mold Dicytostelium. These cells move freely as amoebae on a suitable substrate, but they can suddenly halt their random motions and migrate, as if obeying an invisible command, to a central area where they consolidate into a multicellular organism. This little "snail" migrates across the medium, then raises itself and finally releases spores. This conversion of individual unicellular species into a cell cooperative is most impressive when seen in time-lapse photography. Less theologically inclined biologists spoke of the workings of some substance and gave a name to the God of the amoebae: acrasin, since Dicytostelium belongs to the order Acrasiales. It was only within the last few years that the chemical structure of this compound was elucidated. People had already encountered it repeatedly, however, without knowing it.

In the 1950's it was discovered that glycogenolysis in liver cells is regulated by a low-molecular-weight, heat stable substance, adenosine-3′,5′-monophosphate, or cyclic AMP for short. This special nucleotide is prepared from ATP by an enzyme localized in the cell surface:

$$\text{ATP} \xrightarrow[\text{cyclase}]{\text{adenyl}} \text{cAMP} + \text{pyrophosphate}.$$

Adrenalin favors this reaction, for instance, and so it is understandable why adrenalin also promotes glycogenolysis. Hence, cAMP has been designated as an executive arm of this hormone, and is often spoken of as a "secondary messenger" (E. Sutherland). It has since turned out that not only adrenalin has an "errand boy", but so do other hormones such as glucagon, adrenocorticotropic hormone, and melanocyte stimulating hormone. In each case cAMP was the secondary messenger. On top of this now came the surprising discovery that Acrasin, which causes the asocial single cells of Dicytostellium to join to build a multicellular organism, is nothing other than cAMP.

In the last few years cAMP has become probably one of the most cited and discussed compounds around. Its possibilities of controlling biological processes seem inexhaustible. Somewhat ironically, but accurately, a correspondent for Nature could thus remark: "For those persons who regret the passing of vitalism, the nearest thing to the *élan vital* is nowadays cyclic AMP."

It is obvious that cyclic AMP could also be tried in tumor therapy, and the example of the Acrasiales suggests the thought that the social behavior of other cells could also be influenced. In fact it has already been reported that the "God of the amoebae" could influence the growth of tumors in vitro as well as in vivo. Of course, it is intuitively obvious that a substance that can act in so many cells can be introduced into tumor therapy only with very special precautions.

Summary

Attack on the DNA of a tumor cell stands at the forefront of tumor therapeutic models: using *antimetabolites,* the wrong building blocks are introduced, or synthesis of the correct ones is blocked. *Alkylating agents* simply "hammer away" at the completed DNA.

Asparaginase works more gently: it starves tumor cells by catabolizing the asparagine essential for them.

The basic principle of *multistep* therapy is to set off the natural cytolytic mechanisms, but strictly localized in the cancer tissue.

Antiviral remedies may work preventively, but should not be expected to have an effect on a gross tumor.

DOGMAS OF TUMOR INDUCTION

In his "Maghrebinischen Geschichten," Gregor von Rezzori tells the story of a certain Schorodok and his rain theory. "Rain comes from clouds," this man says. "But the clouds are like sponges soaked with water. Now these soaked sponges are driven across the sky by the wind. Sponges come from the right, sponges come from the left, they meet in the middle and are squeezed together. But if you squeeze a sponge that's full of water, the water comes out of the sponge. It falls to earth, and that's why it rains." Now if one were so brash as to ask for proof of this theory, Schorodok answered, "What proof do you need? Don't you see that it's raining?"

Theory and observation, hypothesis and experiment are not always tied up so loosely as in this example. But there is no science without premature proposals or even prejudices, and cancer research is no exception. This science in particular, with its widely scattered observations, with its confusing isolated observations, in fact needs vigorous prejudices to hack the initial trail through the impenetrable jungle of apparently irreconcilable facts and concepts.

Still it is not pure fantasy that has developed these ideas: people started with good hard data. Warburg had measured respiration and glycolysis again and again before he brought out his cancer theory of deranged respiration. The Millers and Potter had observed the binding of carcinogens to proteins and seen that these proteins were lacking in the resulting tumors. Only then did they formulate the deletion hypothesis. K. H. Bauer had paid close attention to the mutagenic and carcinogenic effects of X-rays before he worked out a general "mutation theory of cancer." Oberling had studied virus tumors thoroughly before writing that tumor viruses must be the cause of all tumors.

Scientific prejudices are destined for revision, at least in principle. But in reality they have as durable a life span as all prejudices and many of them are never really shown to be wrong; they just get old and lose their attraction. "Old soldiers never die, they just fade away." The heat of discussion slowly evaporates, but often not without a certain pang of farewell.

In the daily life of science there are vital, mostly unspoken prejudices, small-change dogmas for daily use. Many of them have slipped into the realm of the "obvious," but it is worth dusting them off from time to time and testing their basic credibility.

Not All Tumor Cells Grow Faster

A few cells of a virulent tumor can become a growth of several grams within a few days: a Novikoff hepatoma or a Yoshida sarcoma kills a rat about a week after transplantation. It is rather immaterial whether the tumor cells develop into a solid growth or multiply as free individual cells (ascites tumor) in the peritoneal cavity. In these cases tumor cells really behave like bacteria in a nutrient-rich medium: they are dedicated almost exclusively to the business of dividing. Even when slowly growing tumors gradually overrun their mother tissues, the tumor cells are growing faster than their normal neighbor.

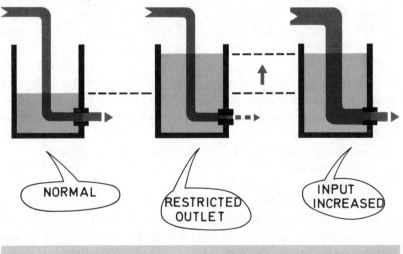

NORMAL   RESTRICTED OUTLET   INPUT INCREASED

HYDRODYNAMIC MODEL OF TUMORGROWTH

Figure 47

But the generalization that all tumor cells divide faster is false. Consider a hydrodynamic model (Figure 47): a constant fluid level is maintained in a vessel; input and output are the same. If the level is to be increased, either the input can be increased or the output can be throttled down. Both cases result in an unstable situation; the content of the vessel has to increase. (Of course, in our model the water level cannot continue to increase indefinitely: as the water level increases, so does the pressure and consequently the exit pressure. At some new level the rate of output equals the increased input rate. Thus the water level is pegged at a new value.)

Nor does tumor growth necessarily have to be maintained exclusively by increased cell division. A lengthening of the mean life span of the individual cells accomplishes the same thing.

In the example of keratinizing skin cells, it could be observed that neoplastic cells live longer than normal cells, and that the processes of normal aging and the transition into "dead" keratin layers are considerably slowed. Such an overaged cell population must necessarily increase in mass. Setälä has spoken of "defective cell maturation" in this connection, as opposed to the alternative of "accelerated cell division."

Epidermal tumors are not the only examples of tumors that can develop at the outset without increased mitoses. In leukemic cell populations, too, there are "eternally young" cells that do not want to make room for the lymphocytes coming behind.

Hence, not all tumor cells grow faster.

Dogma of Transformation

This dogma says: "Carcinogens, be they chemical substances, physical influences, or oncogenic viruses, convert normal cells into tumor cells" (Figure 48).

At first glance this thesis is immediately obvious, and it is an unspoken assumption behind many biochemical investigations of carcinogenesis. On closer examination, however, one must admit that carcinogens attack whole tissue and not individual cells.

Until recently, the tumor viruses were the only "carcinogens" that could transform a normal cell by direct attack. Only in the last few years has it become possible to transform tissue culture cells with chemical carcinogens in vitro (Sachs, Heidelberger, and others).

Dogma of Transformation

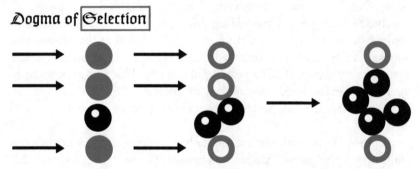

A carcinogen transforms a normal cell to a neoplastic cell, which leads to a new cell population no longer subject to the rules of growth regulation.

Dogma of Selection

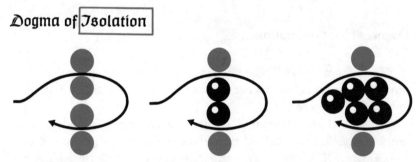

A carcinogen selects preexisting tumor cells; toxic "side effects" of carcinogens on normal cells play the deciding role here.

Dogma of Isolation

A carcinogen separates normal cells from the growth regulatory field. In extreme cases, completely normal cells can behave "neoplastically."

Figure 48

Still, these experiments do not *prove* that carcinogenic agents convert normal cells directly into tumor cells *in the whole animal*. In fact, indications are piling up that indirect mechanisms in carcinogenesis are not to be underestimated. But this brings us to the next dogma.

Dogma of Selection

This dogma says: "Carcinogens select pre-existing tumor cells; they do not induce new tumor cells" (Figure 48).

This dogma assumes that tumor cells are more resistant to toxic carcinogens than normal cells. There is in fact experimental evidence for this:

1. Normal liver cells are poisoned by carbon tetrachloride; extensive necroses form in the liver parenchyma. Cells of a carbon tetrachloride-induced tumor, however, are largely resistant to the necrotizing effects of this solvent.

2. Fibroblasts in tissue culture are injured by benzpyrene. Cells from benzpyrene-induced sarcomas are resistant to this hydrocarbon.

3. Dimethylnitrosamine (DMN) induces liver tumors. Normal liver cells are injured by DMN; extensive necroses can form in the liver. DMN-induced tumors are insensitive to the toxic effect of DMN. Emmelot found an obvious explanation for this resistance: normal liver cells have an enzyme system which converts DMN into its active form ((see page 68). This system is lacking in the resistant tumor cells, and the poisoning by DMN does not occur.

The selective resistance to carcinogens is a rather natural explanation of the overgrowth of a neoplastic cell line within the total population of a tissue. The toxic effect of the carcinogens would thus not be a side effect, but the actual driving force of carcinogenesis. Even in the 1930's Haddow had postulated this, after he had observed that the injurious effects of all of the carcinogenic substances investigated were correlated with their carcinogenic activity.

Of course, all cases in which a short-term administration of carcinogen leads to tumors cause difficulties. If rats receive a half-lethal dose of diethylnitrosamine within a 3-day period, they form kidney carcinomas at 12–14 months. If a high dose (200 μg) of methylcholanthrene is painted on the back of a mouse, papillomas and carcinomas eventually develop. Hamsters die of tracheal papillomas after a single subcutaneous injection of diethylnitrosamine. Finally, the response of mice to promotion by the active fraction of croton oil (A_1) is the same, whether promotion is begun 1 week or 11 weeks after treatment with 25 µg of dimethylbenzanthracene per mouse. It is not quite as easy to see how the carcinogen is supposed to effect a selection in these cases.

But why do the tumors develop so much later? This must be due to processes that no longer have a direct connection with a selective effect of the carcinogen.

One might consider a slow weakening of the organism's defense against the preformed tumor cells. Such decreases in these defense mechanisms with age are well known in immunology. This would mean that the "tumor cells" produced with a one-shot dose must wait for this moment.

The dogmas of transformation and selection are not mutually exclusive. Why shouldn't a carcinogen first transform a cell and then be able to select for it? This might simply be a description of the two-step process of tumor induction. But regardless of whether selection alone or in concert with transformation leads to tumor formation, there are very unpleasant consequences for all investigations concerned with biochemical or histological changes during carcinogenesis.

Consider one example: it has been observed that administration of a carcinogen (methylcholanthrene; dimethylbenzanthracene) is followed by a lowering of DNA synthesis in the tissue (skin), in turn followed by an increase in synthesis. Hence it was concluded that the so-called "primary events" leading to the conversion to a tumor cell have something to do with DNA metabolism. But this conclusion is most hasty, for the observed effects could just as well be the first steps in a reaction chain leading to toxic degeneration of the tissue and not to a tumor cell. The selection dogma would even insist that this has to be so; essentially all carcinogens are toxic, which means that at sufficient dosage they lead to cell damage and in certain cases to cell death.

These toxic "side effects" in tumor induction are familiar to every human pathologist. Inflammation and the appearance of papillomas are closely coupled in the skin; cirrhosis and liver cancer also appear to be directly connected. Cancer never appears in a healthy skin, and there is a similarly poor chance that hepatomas form in healthy liver.

In animal experiments, too, severe liver damage results from feeding hepatotropic substances such as DAB or a few nitrosamines.

At low doses of diethylnitrosamine, however (2 mg/kg/day), hepatomas can be induced *without* liver cirrhosis.

In this case, carcinogenic and toxic effects obviously part company.

It thus appears questionable whether selection alone is really important in tumor induction.

Dogma of Isolation

The dogma of selection made tumor development a simple matter: tumor cells do not have to be formed first; they can be there from the beginning, having appeared during embryonic development. At first they merely lie in the tissue as a harmless little nest; potentially malignant, they wait for their chance.

The dogma of transformation lays the accent decidedly on the role of the individual cell, which is to be converted into a tumor cell by a carcinogen. Logically, then, isolated cells in tissue culture can be transformed by carcinogens in vitro.

But the cells of a higher organism are members of a highly complex community and thus subject to the regulatory impulses of the community existence.

The "dogma of isolation" considers the formation of a tumor from the standpoint of this high placed regulatory field of the whole organism. In a few words: "If cells are separated from growth-regulating signals, they react with neoplastic growth" (Figure 48).

Let us make this concept more apparent with a thought experiment: a liver has been partly removed and is in the process of regrowing. Current theories on liver regeneration depend on liver-regulating substances which are produced by the liver cells themselves and which brake the division of a liver cell, once the liver has again been fully regenerated. The residual liver can naturally produce only a little inhibitor, and the inhibition per individual cell is less:

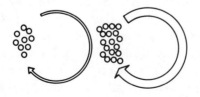

The remaining liver cells can divide, up until about the same number is reached as before the hepatectomy. Then enough liver cells are producing enough liver inhibitor ("chalone"), and division must be shut down.

Now, if the flow of information in this regulatory cycle — liver cells, liver inhibitor — is broken somewhere, the regeneration of the liver would never reach a standstill:

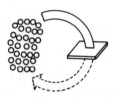

The consequence would be a hepatoma, although a remarkable one, since it would consist of entirely normal liver cells. As yet this example is only a thought experiment. No carcinogen is yet known that specifically reacts with circulating growth regulators and thus shelters a certain tissue from this regulator.

But perhaps the so-called plastic foil sarcomas have something to do with such an interference. These tumors result when, for example, a plastic film is implanted in a rat. Possibly these films then simply interrupt the exchange of regulatory substances.

Oppenheimer had wrapped rat kidneys in cellophane or implanted cellophane foil subcutaneously. It was important how the cellophane was implanted: small rods of the same material with rough surfaces produced no sarcomas. It was concluded therefore that it is not the substance itself that induces the tumor, but a "flow interruption" that it caused in the tissue.

Not only cellophane proved to be carcinogenic. Dozens of other synthetics (polyethylene, polyvinyl, nylon, etc.) led to sarcomas, as did natural polymers such as horn, parchment, or ivory, *if* they were implanted subcutaneously as smooth discs (Druckrey, Schmähl, others).

Of course, it could be shown that the plastic materials did not lie under the skin completely inert. A constant degradation could be shown using radioactively labeled plastics. But the general impression is much more in favor of a "physical," rather than a chemical sarcoma induction. Of course, whether a "chalone equilibrium" is shifted or not is a questionable matter.

The organism surrounds the plastic disc or foil with a capsule of connective tissue, isolates it, and creates an "ecological niche." In fact, the inside of the capsule does act "extraterritorial": cell implants that were rejected elsewhere grow here. The protecting capsule removes the transplanted cells from the attack of the enemy lymphocytes.

Let us consider another example in which isolation and protection obviously play a deciding role in carcinogenesis. Shelton *et al.* placed mouse embryo tissue into a chamber with Millipore walls (semipermeable — to materials smaller than whole cells). These chambers were implanted in the peritoneal cavities of mice (naturally from the same strain) and removed after 14 months. The embryonic tissue was removed and again injected into mice of the same strain, with subsequent formation of sarcomas.

Here again was carcinogenesis by isolation, in this case probably by protection from cellular defense mechanisms. Lymphocytes which would normally do away with small numbers of neoplastic cells could not get into the Millipore chambers. Of course, the question of whether potential tumor cells were present in the embryonic tissue to begin with or arose only because of the "crowded conditions" remains unanswered. But here, too, we are forced to conclude that a carcinogenic agent does not necessarily have to convert a normal cell into a tumor cell which then automatically throws off the shackles of regulation. Obviously, what is decisive here is an indirect effect which leads to collapse of the protecting control mechanisms, without having to directly attack the cells concerned.

Immunosuppression is also connected here: carcinogenic agents injure the immune system, so that preformed or newly formed tumor cells have a better chance of survival. The sheltering Millipore chambers may be mimicking a generally weakened lymphocytic defense system.

Let us consider one last example in which a tumor is induced by isolation of cells. Ovaries can be transplanted into the spleen. In these "splenic ovaries" there first develops a hyperplasia and finally an ovarian tumor. Hence, normal tissue in the wrong place appears to be especially endangered.

Analogous cases are known in descriptive pathology: dispersed tissue of the stomach mucosa can turn up in the esophagus. This "dystopic tissue" also shows a particular tendency to tumor formation. Obviously, stomach mucosa in "Diaspora" can no longer be contacted by the regulating impulses of the mother tissue.

The development of tumors from the splenic ovaries is hormone-conditioned: the estrogen produced by normal ovaries regulates the secretion of gonadotropic hormone (GSH) by the pituitary gland; GSH in turn stimulates cell division in the ovaries. A low level of estrogen effects a large secretion of GSH and the reverse.

The hormone produced in the splenic ovaries goes to the liver, is broken down, and never does reach the pituitary. Hence, the pituitary "thinks" that there are not enough ovary cells; it secretes GSH constantly and the splenic ovaries are thus continually forced to grow.

Transplantability Does not have to be a Criterion of a Tumor

A true tumor must be transplantable. All tumors that owe their existence exclusively to regulatory collapse in the whole organism are thus excluded. If they are transplanted into a new organism that still has intact regulatory mechanisms, they don't have a chance. Strict application of this rule would not recognize growths of the sort of the ovarial tumors in the spleen. But the criterion of transplantability also has its problems with tumors that have removed themselves from the regulatory field of the organism under their own power. Even such "autonomous" tumor cells will only grow when the recipient is immunologically compatible and when they themselves do not evoke too much of a tumor specific immune response. In short, the strict rules of transplantation still hold. A successful take of a tumor thus primarily says something about the immunological relationship of the partners (tumor cell-recipient). Only secondarily does the tumor cell play a role as an autonomous cell.

We still have not exhausted the problems of tumor transplantation as a test for autonomy. Let us compare three closely related examples of transplantation:

1. A transplanted kidney, assuming favorable donor and recipient, grows and functions as a kidney just as it did in its "home organism."

2. Isolated kidney cells transplanted into a syngeneic host do *not* grow.

3. Isolated cells from a kidney tumor *can* be successfully transplanted. They grow into three-dimensional tissues, more or less resembling kidney tissue, with their own vascular networks and surrounded by a protecting capsule. The capsule and the blood vessels were supplied by the host under compulsion from the tumor.

Obviously this "talent for organization" helps to decide whether a tumor cell takes on transplantation or not. Cells might escape from all growth-regulating systems and it would still not be expected that they would have to be transplantable in every case.

Dogma of Irreversibility

"A tumor cell which has once gone the way of anarchy can never be brought back to the path of civil good behavior," according to this dogma. It can be destroyed or rendered harmless, but never be converted back into the normal cell it once was.

Long clinical experience relies on radical attack more than on spontaneous cure. Millions of animal tumors have confirmed this dogma again and again. It has become one of the fundamentals of the mutation theory of cancer, for it is mutations which can explain such irreversible changes.

Still, there is a timid voice of contradiction: in contrast to the overwhelming number of irreversible tumors, the few examples of reversible growths play hardly any role. But just their existence forces a breach in calcified thought systems and necessitates some rethinking.

A. Braun has demonstrated with a plant tumor that tumors *can* be forced to return home. In his experiments he used a tobacco teratoma, a slowly growing tumor that grows on simple, artificial media, is transplantable, and can still produce structures resembling buds and leaves.

A small piece of such a tobacco teratoma was grafted to the cut stem of a healthy tobacco plant. The tumor grew and produced amorphous tissue and also abnormal leaves and buds. If pieces from this growth were again grafted, normal leaves and buds eventually resulted after several passages, and even blossoms were formed. Finally seeds were obtained that gave rise to completely "healed" tobacco plants.

The Viennese Seilern-Aspang and Kratochwil observed tumors in newts which can regress spontaneously. These growths had been induced with methylcholanthrene, they metastasized, infiltrated neighboring tissue until the animals finally died. But in numerous newts the tumor stopped growing and reverted to normal differentiated cells. Tumors that had developed on the tail stump reverted especially easily if regeneration of this part of the body was induced by cutting off the tail.

Possibly the reversibility of this newt tumor is closely connected to the pronounced capability of this animal to regenerate tissue. But it would probably be too pessimistic to see nothing but special rarities in such reversible tumors. Let us look, then, at an example of a mammalian tumor.

So-called teratocarcinomas are known both in mice and men; these are growths consisting of bone, cartilage, and nerve cells, and which also contain hair follicles, the groundwork for teeth, and other differentiated cell types. Besides these specialized cells there are also "embryonic" undifferentiated tumor cells. All of these different cells grow among each other chaotically. A teratoma can be transplanted from mouse to mouse, and the teratoma carrier dies after two to three weeks.

Kleinsmith and Pierce then asked whether each individual cell type had to be transplanted to guarantee the whole spectrum of the teratoma. It turned out to be sufficient to transplant the undifferentiated; all of the other differentiated cell types could develop from them. Here, too, a transition of undifferentiated malignant tumor cells into differentiated cells takes place. No regressions appeared, but this example shows that specialized "normal cells" can very well arise from "embryonic" tumor cells.

Granted, the case of this teratoma is somewhat confusing, but in the meantime reversions have occasionally been observed in other tumor cells of higher organisms. Cells from neuroblastomas lost their undifferentiated appearance after several passages in tissue culture, and more and more resembled normal nerve cells. This is especially odd, since tumor cells in culture normally become *more* malignant, and even normal cells sometimes turn into tumor cells all by themselves in culture.

Sachs recently reported on polyoma-transformed hamster cells of which a high percentage reverted, lost their virulence, or even became "completely normal" again. These reversions can be influenced by variations in culture conditions (low cell density, etc.). The virus genome had *not* disappeared in the reverted cells, but they now contained *more* chromosomes than the starting transformed cells. These observations suggested that the excess chromosomes in the revertants can hold the virus genome in check. This suggestion gains plausibility from experiments performed by Pollack: he was also able to isolate "normal" cells, inhibited by contact, from virus-transformed tumor cells (SV40-3T3), and these revertants also had excess chromosomes.

Sachs took these findings as the occasion to suggest that two types of chromosomes are necessary, one for the expression of malignancy and one for its suppression. In a normal cell these two types are balanced against each other; in a tumor cell the influence of the expression-type predominates. Upon admixture of chromosomes of the suppression type, "normal" cells would again arise out of tumor cells.

The investigations undertaken by Harris on cell hybrids fit into this concept: upon fusion of malignant with normal cells he obtained hybrids that no longer grew as tumor cells and that naturally contained more chromosomes than the starting cells.

Reversible plant tumors, regressing newt cancers, differentiation of embryonic tumor cells in teratocarcinoma, and nerve cells in culture testify against the idea that the deciding difference between a tumor cell and a normal cell is supposed to be a mutation in the genetic material.

The evidence suggests rather that there was only a change in the expression of the cell's genetic potentialities. In their tumorous condition the crown gall tumor cells retained all the factors, genetic and nongenetic, that had been present in the normal state; nothing was lost or permanently rearranged. The cells were made tumorous simply by activation of some of the ordinarily inactive genes; the cells returned to the normal state when these genes were again repressed and rendered nonfunctional (Braun).

Evidence of derepression (although no indication of reversibility) was even found by Baldwin in a rat hepatoma induced by an azo dye. In this tumor he found an antigen identical by immunochemical methods with an antigen from normal rat lung. Finally, a sophisticated model regulatory system has been imagined by Pitot and Heidelberger, who showed how a chemical carcinogen could cause a heritable change without a mutation in the genetic material. They further demonstrated how such an inherited change could revert to the normal state.

But reversibility does not have to mean that an individual cell also reverts. A long time ago Hieger pointed out that "it is the tissue changes which are reversible, there is no evidence that the individual cells themselves are in a reversible equilibrium state." In reversible tumors, normal cells could simply gradually replace the tumor cells.

Dogma of the Reprogramed Tumor Cell

All cells of a higher organism are begotten in the last analysis from one single cell, the fertilized ovum that arose from the union of the maternal ovum with the paternal semen.

Billions of somatic cells arose from this single cell by division; throughout the long process of differentiation they became what they are: kidney cells, nerve cells, liver cells, connective tissue cells. The hereditary material was transmitted to the daughter cells at each cell division: thus each somatic cell has at its disposal the same hereditary material and thus the same DNA as the fertilized egg cell.

Botanists have known this for a long time. If a disc is punched out of a green tobacco leaf and placed in nutrient medium, the piece of green leaf puts down white roots and develops subsequently into a new tobacco plant. The highly differentiated leaf cells must have contained the genetic information necessary for development of a whole plant. In plants, the cultivation of offspring from differentiated somatic cells is nothing unusual. As is their nature, plant cells often remain "multipotent," having the capability to call on their total store of inherited information in an "emergency."

Only recently has it become possible to demonstrate that the somatic cells of animals also have the entire genome of the egg at their disposal. Of course cytogeneticists had long claimed that the hereditary material of the egg was not squandered, but faithfully copied into the daughter cells, but they still had not come up with conclusive proof.

Gurdon of Oxford University attempted this proof: he removed the nucleus from an intestinal epithelial cell of a frog and implanted it in an egg cell of the same species. The nucleus of this egg cell had been "removed" by "killing" with collimated radiation. Operations of this type naturally make a highly subtle surgical technique a prerequisite. The frog's eggs with intestinal nuclei developed into normal tadpoles and finally into normal frogs. Thus it was proved that the somatic cells of a higher animal could still retain the genetic material of the zygote (Figure 49).

It follows that a liver cell or a nerve cell only calls on a limited amount of its genetic information. The residue remains quiet. Today people speak of repression patterns typical for each type of cell: in each cell certain information, i. e., DNA sequences must be uncovered and be "primed." This uncovered material constitutes the program

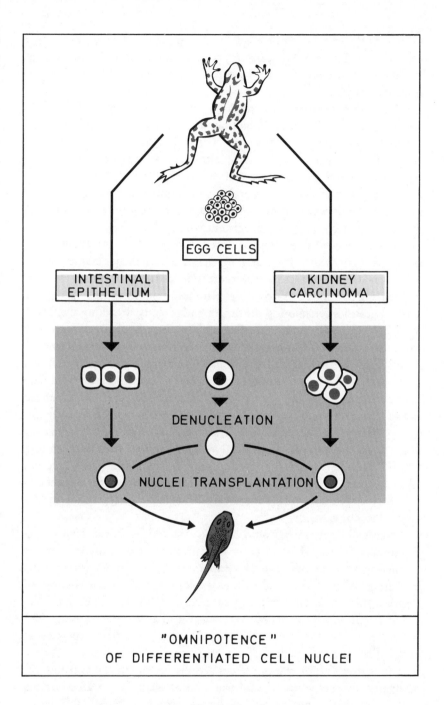

Figure 49

unique to the cell — a muscle cell, a liver parenchymal cell, or a basal cell of the epidermis. There are no mutations on the way from an egg cell to an intestinal cell; otherwise, one could not get intact frogs from intestinal nuclei.

After these preliminary remarks we can now try to formulate another dogma of tumor induction, the dogma of the falsely programed tumor cell: "In principle, the difference between a normal cell and a tumor cell is the same difference as that between a liver parenchymal cell and a nerve cell." The new program of the tumor cell would be sufficiently inexorable to guarantee that, as a rule, only new tumor cells were formed. It would not, however, be so rigid as to exclude reversion, i. e., new program changes.

The dogma of the "reprogramed tumor cell" also furnishes a plausible framework for carcinogenesis: a carcinogen would be a substance that could change a repression pattern, a substance that might "shift" the DNA-covering histones, evoking a new program. The danger of overshooting the target and directly attacking the DNA must be great, and the mutagenic and toxic effects of carcinogens are to be interpreted as just such reactions resulting from overshooting.

We have seen that cell divisions (primarily DNA synthesis) are necessary for the transformation of normal cells into tumor cells. The "new" dogma offers an easy explanation: at each division, or more exactly, at each doubling of DNA of a differentiated cell, the repression pattern must also be copied. Thus DNA synthesis is a "dangerous phase" for the correct transmittal of the detailed directions saying which DNA regions are supposed to remain active and which inactive (the "histone pattern"). The close connection between carcinogenesis and DNA synthesis thus thoroughly "fits" the concept of a reprogramed tumor cell.

A crucial experiment could bring a decision on this dogma in the foreseeable future. If there is no need for the genetic material to be touched in a tumor cell, then the implantation of a tumor cell nucleus into an egg should also lead to the development of a normal embryo. Perhaps this experiment will not succeed on the first try. Perhaps the tumor nucleus will have to be back-transplanted into an egg cell several times before it is again "normalized." The first experiments in this direction will be described later (see page 249).

The cytoplasm of the egg plays a decisive role in the Gurdon experiments, by compelling the information of the differentiated nucleus to "begin at the beginning." Why shouldn't a "neoplastic cytoplasm" also force a nucleus to become a tumor cell nucleus, or why shouldn't a normal cytoplasm lead a tumor nucleus back to normality? The dogma of the reprogramed tumor cell offers the cytoplasm decisive control possibilities. In the "democratic" interplay between nucleus and cytoplasm, there is a consensual decision on the course of the cell.

Summary

Many basic problems in experimental cancer research must still necessarily be decided upon dogmatically.

Thus it is undecided whether

a) A tumor cell can be directly converted into a tumor cell (*transformed*),

b) pre-existing tumor cells are simply *selected*, or

c) somatic cells are simply *isolated* from normal growth regulation.

The discovery of reversible tumors calls into question the assumption that carcinogenesis is fundamentally a "road of no return." The dogma of the reprogramed tumor cell thus compares the difference between a hepatoma cell and a liver cell with the difference between a liver cell and a kidney cell. The new program includes the loss of former capabilities as well as the acquisition of new faculties.

Not all tumor cells grow faster. Occasionally, cells forget to die and increase the population of a tissue in this way.

TUMOR THEORIES IN DIALOGUE

A Fictitious Conversation

Theories without experiments must be blind.
Experiments without theories must remain mute.

"*Ideas, like men, are born, have their adventures, and die,*" the historian of science W. P. D. Wightmann once wrote. Do you believe that this description also applies to the many tumor theories which have come into circulation over the years?

No tumor theory has yet really died. Experimental cancer research is a young science, and consequently there is a whole series of veteran theories that are still fully active. We have a pluralistic society of tumor theories and tumor researchers, with many different opinions, hypotheses, and concepts.

Could you give us an example of an older, still active cancer theory?

A quite odd example would be the "karyogamic tumor theory" of the Frenchman Hallion (1907). Hallion viewed the cause of cancer as a fusion of tissue cells with motile cells such as leukocytes or even bacteria.

> By this act of anarchy, the cell has voided the law to which its normal development is subject. No happening could interfere more disturbingly with the manifestation of the total plan for all cells than an unforeseen and unsuitable fertilization process, which substitutes an abnormal drive to growth for the normal one of the germ cells. The social pact binding the cells is broken, and the independent cell line resulting from this revolutionary act bears the mark of lawlessness as a permanent sign of its unnatural origin and nature.

An entirely Victorian aversion to "amoral cell life" is heard in this formulation, but any kind of proof for this kind of "copulation against nature" was lacking. Almost exactly 50 years later, however, there would be no more doubt that "unnatural copulation" between tissue cells and foreign genetic material is possible and can lead to cancer cells.

You're thinking about tumor viruses?

Yes. Here, the male partner, so to speak, is completely reduced to his naked chromosome, to his naked nucleic acid. But exactly as in a real fertilization, there is a fusion of hereditary material.

Aren't there methods known now for artificially inducing cell fusion?

Yes. True cell hybrids can be obtained using killed Sendai virus. It is conceivable that Hallion's theory could be proved in the near future.

We've already gotten pretty deep into details. Shouldn't we start off this discussion with a simple question: what is cancer?

This is hardly a simple question. We aren't even sure that it's a useful question. Many cancer researchers think that "cancer is connected to the failure of a basic mechanism of life itself" (Oberling). But this would mean that we would have to know what life is before we could understand what cancer is. "The riddle of cancer" would seem to be well hidden, but this is hardly a reason for pessimism. Of course, nobody today knows what life really is, but in the last few decades we have learned more details about living systems than in the preceding centuries. Experimental cancer research simply needs to adopt the recipe for success used in modern biology: eschew general definitions and substitute simple questions that can be approached by experiment.

Is this supposed to mean that experimental cancer research should avoid theories and hyoptheses?

Just the opposite. "Observation is always observation in the light of theories" (Popper), and even biochemical measurements and morphological findings on tumor material remain lifeless data as long as there is no theoretical foundation. "Scientific pronouncements are not derived by pure generalization from observed data, but are constructed as hypotheses" (Bierwisch).

Which theory would you prefer: the chemical, virus, or radiation theory of tumors?

I hate to say this, but none of these examples is a theory. I'll grant you that pathologists occasionally talk about a chemical theory of cancer, but they do this from the standpoint of the autopsy room and the operating table. They try to explain a tumor upon whose appearance they had no influence. For them a tumor is a criminalistic problem, and "chemical tumor theory" simply describes a possibility of how an individual tumor might have arisen. Thus, the "chemical occupational cancers" become separated from the anonymous mass of "spontaneous tumors," as are the radiation cancers of uranium miners or radiologists.

In contrast, experimental cancer research by definition does not recognize spontaneous tumors; tumors that occasionally appear spontaneously are only painful annoyances. Experimental cancer research knows a whole series of procedures for inducing tumors, and in this sense there is no chemical theory of tumors, just chemical recipes for inducing tumors. The same is true for the so-called virus theory: for the tumor virologists there is exact information on which viruses can be used to induce tumors in which animals. Thus, tumor viruses are *not a theoretical possibility* but an *experimental tool*. How tumor viruses actually convert a normal cell into a tumor cell, that is the subject of theories; there are also many theories on how chemical carcinogens actually lead to tumors.

What is a "true tumor theory" supposed to do?

We could cite Warburg here again: "Just as there are many remote causes of the plague — heat, insects, rats — but only one common cause, the plague bacillus, so there are uncounted *remote* causes of cancer — tar, radiation, arsenic, pressure, urethane, sand — but only one *common* cause of cancer, into which all these causes of cancer flow "

Of course, today we would make our formulations less apodictic and considerably more cautious and talk only about the *possibility* of a common cause of cancer. But a "true theory of tumors" would have to inform us as to the nature of such a common cause.

Would you include here the information hypothesis of cancer, according to which cancer represents interference in the flow and content of information?

One shouldn't even talk about a theory in this case; it is nothing but the classic definition of a tumor cell in modern terminology. The

232

"information hypothesis" consequently cannot possibly be false, while a "real" theory must have a possibility of failure.

Virchow's irritation theory would be an honest-to-goodness tumor theory, wouldn't it?

Naturally, because it tried to bring the multitude of causes down to a common denominator, and it failed. This common denominator was chronic irritation: radiation cancer arises after chronic inflammation (radiation dermatitis), or liver cancer always succeeds cirrhosis, according to the experience of human pathologists.

The tissue responds to the constant irritation and tries to compensate. Regenerative processes and increased cell divisions play an important role. At first, regeneration stays under control, until ever-more rapidly growing cell lines develop and finally "true" cancer cells are formed.

Virchow drew his conclusions from clinical observation and was later brilliantly confirmed (at first) by experimental cancer research: Yamagiwa's successful induction of tar carcinomas in the rabbit's ear was really nothing more than an application of Virchow's irritation theory.

But weren't there difficulties soon after?

Yes. Irritating and carcinogenic effects did not by any means always run parallel, nor did the induction of sarcomas always follow a simple irritation. 3,4-Benzpyrene and 1,2-benzpyrene have about the same irritating effect, but only the former is carcinogenic. Another example: hepatomas can be induced without cirrhosis, if diethyl-nitrosamine is fed in low enough doses.

Still, Virchow's theory is correct as a starting point: cancer can be induced by (external) stimuli, and it is immaterial whether inflammatory reactions in particular take place at the onset of tumor formation.

But if we really come up with a general definition of the concept "irritation," then everything fits, even the tumor viruses, and the Virchow theory can't be false.

Careful, now: The genetically derived tumors don't fit the irritation concept. We've seen already that certain tumors, especially in certain strains of mice, appear with the precision of clockwork. Irritation here is entirely dispensable, or to put it the other way around, avoiding irritation doesn't help: anarchy is already programmed into the fertilized egg.

The same is true for the experimentally induced tumor-bearing hybrids from closely related species.

You mean the swordtail hybrids that die of melanomas?

Right. Here the simple mixing-in of foreign genetic material interferes with the normal course of development. This recipe doesn't work only in fish. You remember perhaps that hybrids between different tobacco species can develop tumors.

You mean the crosses between Nicotiana langsdorffii and N. glauca?

Yes. Here, too, there appears to be a simple principle involved: *N. glauca* is an annual, "designed" for rapid growth; *N. langsdorffii* is a perennial, sort of a "harnessed" tobacco plant, designed for stability more than for rapid growth. In the hybrid, then, we get a conflict between stability and growth. Naturally these are only qualitative thoughts, but genetic analyses of repressor systems similar to those of the swordtails will probably be the eventual outcome.

Are there more exceptions to Virchow's irritation rule?

The so-called dysontogenic growths also appear to be exceptions: these growths are remarkable mixtures of normal tissues, in which teeth, hair, and skin can grow in and among each other (teratomas). In a few examples rudimentary heads, with or without a brain, along with feet and toes with nails have been formed ("parasitic fetus"). Starting at this "unfortunate twin brother," it appears that one can draw increasingly complex cases of double formation, leading to Siamese twins and then to identical twins. According to this interpretation, a tumor would be a "luckless and degenerate relative" (Oberling) of the host.

In his embryonic theory of tumor development, Cohnheim even interpreted a cancer cell as a dispersed embryonic cell that has stopped developing for some reason . . .

But which has retained its growth potential . . .

Exactly. In the adult organism the organizing and forming powers of the growing embryo are missing, naturally, and it wouldn't be long until the catastrophe.

Are there experiments which support this theory?

The induction of experimental tumors by implantation of embryonic tissue was not a convincing success. To be sure, by "varying injury" to frog's eggs, teratomas, tumors, and even double monsters were obtained. Here it appears that an inducing stimulus is important for dysontogenic growth.

Which brings us right back to Virchow. Let's take a look once more at an abbreviated list of "tumor-inducing principles" (Table 6). It's always amazing how many different and even dissimilar stimuli can induce tumors.

Just the multiplicity of chemical carcinogens is confusing, but the conclusion that most substances are more or less carcinogenic would be hasty. Extremely small changes in a carcinogenic molecule can extinguish its oncogenic properties. There are strict rules governing carcinogenicity within a series of closely related compounds (compare 3,4-benzpyrene and 1,2-benzpyrene), but there seem to be hardly any rules which hold for more than one class of compounds (compare $CHCl_3$, thiourea, naphthylamine).

Musn't it then appear hopeless to find a common denominator among fundamentally different causes of cancer?

Well, one could subscribe to the opinion that each carcinogenic stimulus "goes its own way" to the neoplasm. Many pathologists think so, since there is not only a variety of circumstances under which tumors can arise, but the appearance of the individual growths vary widely from case to case. Many pathologists consequently refuse to recognize extensive similarities.

Table 6: The Diversity of Carcinogens

Chemical stimuli	
Organic compounds	Mustard gases, epoxides, propiolactone
	Diethylnitrosamine, N-methyl-N-nitrosourethane
	β-Naphthylamine, 2-acetylaminofluorene,
	$\quad N,N$-dimethyl-4-aminoazobenzene
	4-Nitroquinoline- N-oxide
	Thiourea, thioacetamide
	3,4-Benzpyrene, 3-methylcholanthrene
	Stilbestrol, Polyvinylpyrrolidone
Natural products	Aflatoxins (from *Aspergillus flavus*)
	Senecio alkaloids, cycasin
Hormones	Pituitary hormones
Nucleic acids	Tumor virus DNA
Inorganic compounds	Asbestos, nickel dust, lead and beryllium
	compounds

Physical stimuli	
Radiation	X-rays, ultraviolet rays, radioactive isotopes
	(^{60}Co, radium)
Mechanical irritation	Wounding (promotion only?)
Heat	Chronic burns
Polymeric substances	Metal foils, synthetic foils (cellophane, etc.)

Biological stimuli	
Parasites	Bilharzia (Tumor viruses?)
Bacteria	*B. tumefaciens* (Tumor viruses?)
Tumor viruses	DNA viruses: Polyoma, adenovirus
	RNA viruses: Rous sarcoma virus, leukemia
	viruses

But there must be at least one common property of tumor cells: they have all escaped the strict growth regulation of their tissue or organism, regardless of whether they were induced by a virus, a chemical carcinogen, or irradiation.

Naturally, and because of this cancer apears to many as a "quite uniform process . . . and the uniformity of the tumor process directly forces many to the thought of a uniformity in the mechanism of induction" (Oberling).

What is the nature of this "uniformity" supposed to be?

Let's look at two thought models:
1. Every carcinogenic stimulus (physical, chemical, or biological) "marches to a different drummer," to be sure, but arrives at the same target complex in the cell at the end.
2. It is only necessary to assume that basically there is only one single cause of cancer. All other cancer-inducing factors appear only as indirect inducers or accelerators.

Well, then, is there something like a hierarchy of carcinogenic stimuli?

It looks like it. There is a clear distinction between the mode of action of a parasite that induces cancer in only 5 to 10 percent of all cases, and that of a carcinogenic nitrosamine that works 100 percent of the time. Besides this gradation in the certainty of effect, there are temporal differences that cannot be overlooked: feeding with carcinogenic azo dyes leads to hepatomas after about a 6-month latent period, while tumor growth begins immediately upon infection with polyoma virus. Certainty of effect and rate of tumor formation would thus be factors recommending tumor viruses as the real cause of cancer.

But in principle then wouldn't cancer have to be contagious?

This nonsense comes up again and again: cancer can't be caused by viruses, since it is not contagious. There is a decisive error here.

Even an infectious disease is not always contagious. Herpes of the lips or shingles are caused by viruses, but they are not contagious. Typhus is one of the most murderous diseases to afflict the human race, but a typhus patient without lice is no more contagious to others than a cancer patient. Most objections to the virus theory are based on an insufficient knowledge of general virology. Many simply cannot be persuaded from the opinion that pathogenic bacteria or viruses always cause disease immediately and under all circumstances. The enormous importance and distribution of latent infections are mostly ignored (Oberling).

Now would this mean that, say, radiation could activate such latent viruses?

It has long been known that irradiation can promote virus infections: Herpes can be activated by sunlight.

Kaplan found that latent tumor viruses too can be activated by X-rays. He irradiated C 57/BL mice with X-rays and obtained lymphomas. Cell-free extracts from these tumors induced tumors of the same type. More exacting analysis of these X-ray-virus leukemias is very complicated (splenic factors, role of bone marrow), but these experiments do show 1) that latent infections are also possible with tumor viruses, and 2) that classical carcinogenic agents such as X-rays occasionally produce tumors via an intermediary.

Well, can chemical carcinogens also dramatize some virus infections?

Surely. Duran-Reynals induced an outburst of fowl pox in chickens by painting with methylcholanthrene. The actual causative virus was obviously already present in the skin in a latent form before the activation.

But whether chemical carcinogens can also "awaken" latent tumor viruses is questionable . . .

Was questionable, we have to say now. Using methylcholanthrene, urethane, and diethylnitrosamine, in mice, Huebner and others could induce lymphomas from which leukemia virus-containing extracts could be prepared.

But this is an isolated observation, at least for the moment.

Yes. Then, too, it was done on the same strain of mice (C 57/BL) in which "symbiotic" tumor viruses can be activated with X-rays. But the indications are increasing that latent tumor viruses are more widespread than oncologists have been willing to admit. Virologists have continually run across the so-called C-particle in the electron microscope. As a start these can be considered to be the same as tumor viruses, since such renowned oncogenic viruses as the Gross leukemia virus and the Rous sarcoma virus are in this class.

The revealing antigenic traces of tumor viruses have been discovered in animal strains and species that previously had been considered to be free of viruses. Among those animals that can be said to be new to tumor research, the cat with its leukemia viruses is the most prominent.

Aren't these the same viruses that also cause leukemia in mice?

They are the same type. But cats are more exciting than mice, not because they are that much more similar to humans, but because as domestic animals they could be an important "environmental factor" in human disease. Occasionally, C-particles have even been demonstrated in human tumor material.

But not regularly.

That isn't at all important; by definition, latent viruses do not always have to be evident. There are recent experiments which indicate that leukemia viruses in particular very probably can exist "fully submerged."

Todaro and coworkers could isolate stable cell lines from mouse embryos of the Balb/c inbred strain, which inoculated into mice of the same strain induce tumors. Real tumor cells had arisen from apparently normal mouse embryo cells via cell culture (rapid passage at high cell densities).

That isn't all that surprising. The induction of malignant cells by simple in vitro culture has often been reported.

The surprising part in this case was that these in-vitro-induced tumor cells produced mouse leukemia virus. The cultivation in vitro obviously had the same effect as the carcinogen treatment in C 57/BL mice: in both cases leukemia viruses were activated.

Couldn't there have been just an accidental virus infection?

Chance infection of the cultures with leukemia virus seems to be excluded. The authors prefer the interpretation that the mouse cells contained the information for a leukemia virus in a completely repressed form. Thus, we would have to add the completely "mute" virus genome to the "phenomenology" of tumor viruses. Huebner speaks of "virogenes," to signify that these viruses really act more like cellular genes and not as infectious agents. True infection between cells obviously does not play an especially important role; propagation of the various viruses can take place completely mute in the vertical mode, from mother cell to daughter cell, and correspondingly from mother animal to offspring.

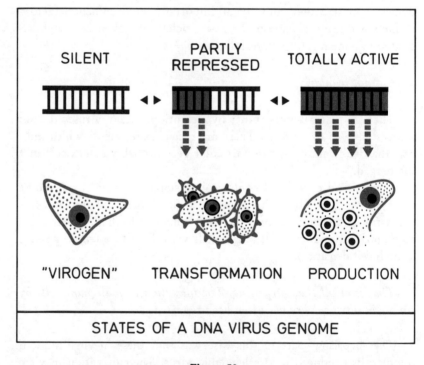

STATES OF A DNA VIRUS GENOME

Figure 50

If I have understood you correctly, the general virus tumor theory is again much talked about. Up until just a year or two ago, there was a completely different impression: arguments weighed heavily against the generalization that all tumors are, in the last analysis, virus tumors.

One of these arguments was supplied by modern tumor immunology: chemically induced tumors possess antigens specific for each tumor. This antigenic individuality even goes so far that two tumors induced in the same animal have different antigens. In contrast, tumors induced by a given virus have been observed always to have the same tumor antigens.

How is this dilemma to be resolved?

It wasn't really so surprising that all tumors induced by the same virus showed the same antigens. Only the monstrous variety in the chemical tumors was astonishing. But why shouldn't there be weaker group specific antigens from tumor viruses among the individually specific antigens of the chemically induced tumors? The variety of strong individual antigens would then cover up a uniform pattern of weak virus antigens. In fact, there has been talk very recently about common "weak" antigens in chemically induced tumors, too.

The variety of different antigens in chemically induced tumors would then no longer seriously stand in the way of a general virus theory. But doesn't the objection still hold that chemical carcinogenesis follows exact quantitative dose-response laws that can have nothing to do with a virus infection?

With a virus infection, no, but very probably with activation of a latent virus within a cell. Carcinogens and time change, if you wish, the growth-regulating parts of a cell, and we have thoroughly discussed these "multihit reactions." But why shouldn't it be just as "tiring and time-consuming" to "dig out" a latent virus?

All in all, you think that the idea that oncogenic viruses represent the real cause of cancer is still entirely attractive and that all other cancer-inducing stimuli can be entered into the group of virus-activating factors. But proof for these ideas is as meager as it ever was, isn't it?

Of course, there is no proof. Involved proponents however have often thought that "it is hard to believe that processes resulting in essentially similar changes of the cell might be induced once by a change in the genetic information of the cell proper, while in other instances by additional genetic information received by the cell from the outside" (Zilber).

Logically, to be sure, it would be no problem to imagine that greatly varying causes can have the same effects . . .

Certainly not. A geneticist would say that different genotypes can give rise to the same phenotype.

Let's just get back to the list of the many causes of cancer. Wouldn't it be simpler to forget about a common denominator?

Naturally. What are X-rays, azo dyes, plastic implants, and polyoma virus supposed to have in common? It would be an obvious solution, that all carcinogenic stimuli only set in motion processes which the cell could carry out without them. The carcinogens would only give the impetus, and the cell can take over from there.

"The explanation (of the cancer problem) is accordingly to be sought in the cell, and not so much in the carcinogen," Lettré writes along these lines. He thinks that "a cell that is to survive a certain degree of damage can parry with only a limited number of forms still fit for life. One of these possible forms is the cancer cell."

Surely this idea isn't new.

No. The idea that carcinogenic stimuli really only liberate latent potentialities was part of the thought behind Virchow's irritation theory: the tissue "responds" to the carcinogenic impulse, and this response prepares the appearance of tumor cells. Not only the "action" of a carcinogen, but the "reaction" of the cell is decidedly important. In other words, normal cells are in an unstable equilibrium.

Similar thoughts are in Warburg's theory of cancer induction: there cancer is apostrophied as a regression to primitive growth habits. Cancer cells again behave like primitive one-celled organisms without social engagement. It is really not so tremendously important whether the newly won glycolysis is solely responsible for this asocial behavior or whether it is only one parameter — essential, of course — of many that belong to this "primitive form of life."

So a tumor cell doesn't learn anything new? It just resurrects old potentialities?

You could put it that way. In this connection you often hear of the "return to the embryonic cell type," to a cell type distinguished by vigorous growth.

In fact, tumor cells lose many functions characteristic for adult tissue and thus resemble the embryonic tissues that have not yet developed these functions. Besides this loss of specific functions, long-forgotten embryonic properties can reemerge in tumor cells. There have been multiple reports of "new tumor antigens" that were nothing more than "old" embryonic antigens, reminiscences of earlier periods of frequent cell divisions.

To be sure, superficial similarities shouldn't mislead us into seeing agreements in basic principles. Foulds once clearly warned us against this, saying: "The relationship between embryonic cells and 'anaplastic' neoplastic cells is much the same as that between a child and a senile man in second childhood; in the one potentialities are undeveloped and in the other they are gone forever."

Because of this, though, similarities do exist — frequent cell division and renunciation of specific functions. Many tumor theories consequently start from the idea that a cell in principle can pendulum between two ground states, viz., cell differentiation and cell division.

Could you be a bit more specific?

This simply means that a cell either divides or carries out "differentiated" functions: for instance, as liver cells store glycogen, prepare blood sugar, and produce bile pigments, or as nerve cells put out long dendrites to neighboring nerve cells.

There is genetic information for each "state," and thus the transition from a differentiated cell to a dividing cell can be imagined as follows: in a cell which is say, part of regenerating liver, differentiated genes are shut off and the gene parts necessary for division are called upon.

But this transition would be reversible, for upon completion of regeneration, further division stops. In contrast, a tumor cell would be a cell that has given up its differentiated functions for good and dedicated itself permanently to the business of division. In Bullough's words, "differentiation collapses into cancer." The "differentiated genes" become dumb, and the genes required for mitosis are transferred to a state of permanent alarm. H. Busch has proposed the name "tumor genes" for these genes.

This concept of a "cancer gene" is quite evident, isn't it?

Only without further consideration. The simple alternative: differentiation or division is obviously a false abstraction. For example, if collagen-producing cell cultures are synchronized and the collagen production followed over the entire cell cycle, no interruption of production is found during the S-phase or even during actual mitosis. Hence, mitosis and differentiated function are not necessarily mutually exclusive.

Don't the minimal deviation hepatomas also show that the tumor property and differentiated function in principle are not mutually exclusive?

Yes. There is a whole spectrum of these hepatomas that grow more or less rapidly and are still more or less clearly reminiscent of liver tissue. The slowly growing ones especially still make glycogen and can even produce bile pigments, both really privileges of a normal liver cell. Thus, here tumor growth is compatible with differentiated functions. "With the advent of experimental tumours of "minimum-deviation" type, the idea that a given cell has two alternative fates — to multiply or to differentiate — has become a rather unprofitable line of though (E. Reid)."

Still, the "cancer gene" concept doesn't have to be wrong, does it?

No. The blockage of "mitosis information" can be disturbed even without having to touch specific functions. Normally, however, the specific functions of a cell are definitely attacked; as a rule, tumor cells can do less than normal cells.

This is really the substance of the deletion hypothesis, which "in its simplest form is intended to mean that a cancer cell lacks some enzyme that is present in the normal cell from which it was derived" (Potter).

How did this hypothesis come about?

It was formulated by the Millers, after they had observed that carcinogens are bound to defined proteins in the cell (h-proteins). In the "finished" tumor cell, these proteins that initially had reacted with the carcinogens are absent.

But h-proteins surely aren't the only things missing in a tumor cell?

Of course not. Usually whole enzyme catalogues are absent, which naturally brings up the question, which of these "deletions" are strategically important deletions? That is, which of them really have something to do with the neoplastic properties of a tumor cell.

Certain changes can be considered to be simply toxic damages, since carcinogens, as we have seen many times, are mostly rather injurious agents, which unavoidably lead to cell death at high dosages.

Can't the "toxic" changes that have nothing to do with carcinogenesis be recognized as such?

The separation of toxic from carcinogenic effects has been tried many times by comparing chemically related substances in their effect on cell metabolism. This makes sense only when the two substances have about the same toxicity. Whatever extra could be done by the compound that was also carcinogenic would then be considered to be specific for carcinogenesis.

We are concerned not simply with the question, toxic or carcinogenic, but also with the problem of whether the conceivable changes in a tumor cell are primary or secondary events, and this question, too, is very difficult to answer. We are already acquainted with chromosome changes that probably arise only as a consequence of precipitate cell divisions and are not their cause. But other parameters could also be changed only subsequently.

Haven't there been occasional attempts to distinguish primary from secondary events, by doing exact temporal analysis and hoping that strategically important events precede secondary events?

Such considerations have been advanced, but another method promises more success in separating the wheat from the chaff: tumors from the same parent tissue are compared and attempts made to establish common properties. Tumors that are especially suited for this are those least different from their tissue of origin (minimal deviation tumors). A short statement of the principle behind such a comparison is as follows: obviously none of the capabilities of these tumors hinders neoplastic growth. If a certain enzyme is lacking in some tumor but is present in a minimal deviation tumor, then it really can't have anything to do with carcinogenesis. Thus, the greatest service of this method is to "demythologize," and many a deletion has already fallen victim to it (especially Warburg's glycolysis).

Are conclusions of this sort really conclusive?

You would like to be careful with "demythologizing" and you're right: let's imagine that three partners in a reaction cycle are necessary for growth regulation of a normal cell:

The deletion (loss) of one of these partners, whether A, B, or C, would put this regulation out of action. The conclusion that the remaining components have nothing to do with regulation would obviously be completely false.

Then would the comparison between minimal deviation tumors permit any certain statements?

It appears not. But if we assume that a single decisive change in a cell is enough to derail it, then comparative investigations do make sense. Granted, a cell is a very complicated network of intertwined cyclic processes. Despite this fact, there is a certain hierarchy: if there is a growth-regulating factor, then it certainly carries more weight for tumor properties than any "peripheral events" in metabolism. In the discussion of the chalone concept we have already become acquainted with such an essential factor.

Let's get back to the question of strategic changes in connection with the deletion hypothesis. Carcinogens react with certain proteins, inactivate them, and then provide for permanent elimination of these substances. But these proteins, if they are important for carcinogenesis, can't be just any proteins, can they?

No, of course not. They would have to be regulator proteins; today we would probably say chalone, to use Bullough's description. But this doesn't solve the problem; how is a temporary inactivation, let's say of a chalone, supposed to lead to its permanent loss? We could ask: how is this *acquired characteristic inherited?*

Inheritance of acquired characteristics is in the twilight of biology now. Lamarck was stricken down by Darwin with no comparable replacement, so how does experimental tumor research solve this problem?

To clear up this "Lamarckian dilemma," Pitot and Heidelberger proposed a double repression cycle of the Jacob-Monod type, which has as its end effect the permanent cessation of synthesis of the "carcinogen-damaged" regulator (repressor). No irreversible change in the actual genetic material is necessary. Theoretically, by addition of intact regulator, the "vicious cycle" would be broken, and the cell could again produce regulator by itself. Accordingly, cancer would be reversible in principle.

If we refer back to Lamarck, why not to Darwin? A cell which has "invented" a double-repressor regulatory cycle like that during evolu-

tion has done itself more harm than good. The "injurious" action of the carcinogen is monstrously dramatized; instead of a temporary loss of regulator, the cell has to do without it permanently. It's throwing the baby out with the bath.

The Pitot-Heidelberger theory has occasionally been called "highly sophisticated," although some workers consider such a description charitable. Still, this theory removes a decisive defect from the protein deletion hypothesis, namely that the simple loss of even a regulator protein cannot lead to a tumor cell. This loss has to be registered with the genetic material of the cell, and the theory shows how this registration can be accomplished.

Doesn't it bother you that the changes should be reversible? Are tumor cells not irreversibly tumor cells?

Yes, it's the sad experience of human medicine and of experimental cancer research that the path to the tumor is a route of no return, overwhelmingly, anyway; this has led to the mutation theory of cancer, and this theory still has a special place today.

Is there any alternative at all to the mutation theory? A tumor cell always leads to a tumor cell, the tumor properties have to be transmitted, and how is that supposed to happen without altered genetic material?

In the broadest sense, every tumor cell is inded a mutated cell, if by that you mean any hereditary change, but this does not mean that the tumor cell also has to be irreversibly changed. Kidney cells normally give rise only to kidney cells, and liver cells to liver cells, without there having to be a genetic difference between them. There is no mutation that distinguishes a kidney cell from a liver cell, and there is no more reason for there to be a mutation distinguishing a liver cell from a hepatoma cell.

What does distinguish a liver cell from a kidney cell?

Simply that in a liver cell different genes are active from those in the kidney cell. In a liver cell, certain parts of the DNA are covered which are open in a kidney cell, and vice versa. The differences then are differences in the "repression pattern" and not differences in primary genetic material.

So you see an alteration in the repression pattern as an alternative to the mutation theory. Do you think that a "reprogramming" can lead to a tumor cell?

Many oncologists think about such program changes, among them Sidney Weinhouse, who has studied glycolytic enzymes in minimal deviation hepatomas. He thinks that a switch in read-out of the genes is involved, so that enzymes that are part of the equipment of a normal liver cell are suppressed, while others that are normally blocked come to the surface.

Such switching could be reversible. Hence, it is of special interest that there obviously appear to be cases of reversible tumors.

Are you thinking about tobacco tumors and the like?

Yes, but also about old experience with bronchial carcinomas. It turned out that many bronchial carcinomas produce ACTH, a protein hormone that is normally not produced in bronchial cells. Obviously, something in these tumor cells which is normally asleep has "awakened."

Has it been generally proved that the highly differentiated cells of an animal still possess the entire genetic material of the fertilized egg?

Don't you remember the experiments done by Gurdon? These were experiments in which he produced whole tadpoles and even frogs by implanting the nuclei from differentiated intestinal cells into egg cells (with killed nuclei). Thus, the intestinal nuclei had contained all of the information necessary for development of a normal adult organism.

If a tumor cell is really only "reprogrammed," then wouldn't a normal frog also have to be produced by implanting a tumor cell nucleus into an egg cell?

R. C. McKinnell and his coworkers have done such experiments: they induced kidney tumors in the frog *Rana pipiens,* isolated nuclei from the tumor, and transplanted them into denucleated eggs. As in the case of the "normal" intestinal cell nuclei, here, too, viable tadpoles developed. Thus, the tumor cell nuclei had retained the information for a whole series of specialized cell types. "Ciliated epithelium propelled the tadpoles in the culture dishes. The tadpoles swam when stimulated. Functional receptors, nerve tissue, and striated muscle are necessary for swimming. Cardiac muscle pumped blood cells through external gills. The multipotency of the tumor genome was thus obvious before histological examination of the transplant tadpole" (Figure 49).

Doesn't this conclusively refute the idea that a tumor absolutely has to be a mutated cell?

Not yet. The deciding mutation would really have to be expressed only in adult kidney cells, and the tadpoles have not been brought to that stage yet. Besides, we have to remember that the original tumor was a virus tumor, and it would be entirely reasonable if the virus genome were simply to be lost upon the implantation into the egg cell. Thus, we would have to wait and see if chemically induced tumors behave similarly. But the idea of a "reprogrammed" cell has increased in plausibility, without doubt.

Could we consider the cytoplasm of an egg cell to be a "fountain of youth" for differentiated nuclei?

Fountain of youth or not, the cytoplasm has a role in the decisions of a cell in any case. This cooperative decision making doesn't stop at the nuclear membrane.

It is not absolutely necessary to transplant a differentiated cell nucleus into an egg cell to "rejuvenate" it. Harris fused a chicken erythrocyte (which normally doesn't divide any more) with a rapidly dividing tissue culture cell. In this "heterokaryon" there was a visible alteration in the erythrocyte nucleus; it swelled and again took up the DNA synthesis which it had shut off. In short, a cell nucleus was reactivated.

Hasn't the reverse also been observed: suppression of specific cell functions by cell fusion?

Yes. Ephrussi has described such a case: he "crossed" a melanin-producing cell with a melanin-free cell and obtained hybrids without melanin synthesis. His interpretation: in a melanin-free cell, melanin synthesis is suppressed, and the same "repressor" then blocks pigment production in the double cell.

Wouldn't this mean that, in a fusion of a tumor cell with a normal cell, the "neoplastic properties" would have to be lost?

Right. Whatever is missing in the tumor cell (deletion) would be contributed by the partner in the twinned cell. Harris has actually observed such hybrids of tumor and normal cells that had lost their ability to grow as a tumor cell. Others, however, have seen just the opposite: their tumor-normal hybrids were still tumor cells.

Doesn't this contradict the deletion hypothesis?

Only on first appearances, from the perspective of the growth regulator: the bred-in normal cell would have had to be able to supply it. It looks different when we consider the (hypothetical) receptor for this regulator. If this receptor no longer reacts to the regulator in the tumor cell, why should it react in the cell hybrid?

The loss of a regulator or of a receptor for a regulator could be described by a true mutation. But you think that the loss can be explained "simply" by an alteration in the repression pattern, i. e., with a "reprogramming"?

I would even say, possibly, that it is preferable to think of a shift in repression pattern and not of a mutation. But this is not to say that the decisive changes have to take place in the genetic material of the cell at all. Alterations in the DNA hardly exhaust the possibilities one could imagine: a competitor of the mutated nuclear gene required by the classical mutation theory would be the plasma gene, genetic material outside of the nucleus. Autonomous mitochondria would be an example of such plasma genes.

Hasn't there also been speculation about autonomous cell membranes?

In this case "autonomous" cannot mean complete independence from the nucleus, but only a freedom of choice in assembling membrane structural components into specific patterns. Yes, there is such speculation.

Do these "secondary inheritance mechanisms" play any significant role in cancer research today?

Not really. Their greatest value lies in warning against considering the all too obvious theories as theoretical necessities and thus as proved.

We have now rather thoroughly discussed how a tumor cell can remain a tumor cell. Could we now tack on the question of how a normal cell becomes a tumor cell to begin with?

I hope you aren't fishing for a definition: Virchow once thought that "no one, even if he were stretched on the rack, could say what a tumor cell really is." But we could try to give a tentative definition: in the simplest sense, a cell would be a tumor cell when it divides more rapidly than the same cells in its neighborhood.

That would mean that we would have to ask how such unwanted cell divisions are prevented in the normal case.

Yes, but we can only give a general answer to the question. The regulatory fields of the organism are responsible. Purely formally, regulation can be disturbed in two ways: 1) weakening of the regulatory field, or 2) loss of the cell's antennae toward the regulatory field.

These fields could be of *hormonal* nature (as an example). You remember the hormone-dependent mammary carcinomas in mice and rats.

How does the immune system qualify as a regulatory field?

It is assumed, really, that the host's immune defense system goes into action only when tumor cells are already there. It would therefore be regulation after the fact. Of course, the opinion has occasionally been expressed that the immune mechanisms participate directly in the constancy of tissue, for instance by recognizing "senile" cells and carrying them off.

Would simple hindering of the immune response then lead to the appearance of "tumor cells"?

Theoretically, yes, and chemical carcinogens could simply be blocking the removal of dangerous tumor cells by their immunosuppressive effect ("indirect chemical carcinogenesis by immunosuppression").

Is there experimental proof?

We could cite experiments by Stutman: he investigated different strains of mice and found that, in a strain which reacted strongly to methylcholanthrene, the immune system was extensively paralyzed by this hydrocarbon. In another strain which showed hardly any response, the immune capacity was hardly reduced. Hence, tumor formation and immunosuppression appear to be correlated.

Such impressive differences could not be demonstrated in other systems: the induction of lung adenomas, for instance, using methylcholanthrene or urethane, is reduced in thymectomized (= hindrance of immune response) animals, but not eliminated (Trainin).

Then this would mean that immunity effects do not play a role in the actual induction of tumor cells, but can play a very important role in the multiplication of tumor cells already present.

Exactly. It is now generally maintained that immunological effects must be studied to understand the appearance of tumors. Passive immunization of tumor-bearing animals with autologous tumor cells supports this opinion, as do the numerous experiments recently performed with antilymphocytic serum. Again and again, a shortening of the latent periods because of this immune-blocking reagent has been observed, in complete agreement with the idea that immune reactions normally put off the formation of tumors.

Let's complete our list of the regulatory fields set above the cells. Haven't we overlooked the most important one?

Yes. The most important regulatory field might be the tissue itself. For the moment we can leave open the question of whether this field is represented by contact-mediated impulses between cells (possibly even of electrical nature) or by regulatory substances produced in the tissue (chalones).

Shouldn't we attempt one more definition and say something to the effect that tumor cells have become "deaf" to growth-regulating influences. According to the current state of priorities, your opinion would be that they are primarily deaf to the regulatory impulses of their own tissue.

Here, too, we again have to consider two limiting cases of interference with regulation: a) either the cell produces no more regulatory signals (chalones), or b) it can no longer receive signals because it has lost the necessary antennae for them. A cell without antennae would have become a tumor cell automatically.

A cell that can no longer produce signal substances but still reacts to them would be a remarkable tumor cell, wouldn't it?

At first it isn't even recognizable as a tumor cell, as long as it is supplied with sufficient quantities of regulatory substances by its neighbors in the tissue organization. It would have to divide more or less in the rhythm of the normal tissue as a tumor cell incognito, until a nest of cells has grown large enough that it can no longer be supplied with the necessary regulatory substances. Only when this nest of cells has reached a "critical mass" could it then, at least in its inner regions, grow uninhibited.

Isn't the problem of defining a tumor cell primarily complicated by the fact that tumor cells in general have a developmental history?

This is in fact an aggravating difficulty: a tumor cell is by no means definable only statically. It must also be realized as a historical event. Its *history* begins at the point when it escapes the regulatory impulses of its tissue. This step can be described as a loss of normal properties. But a tumor cell of this type can exist only within a well-organized tissue, in which nutrients are brought in and supporting tissue is at hand. If the tumor cell really wants to become autonomous, it must take care of itself. It must induce supporting tissue (stroma) and construct its own vascular system. Without these accomplishments there could be no transplantable tumors.

Then in this phase the tumor cell seems to learn something "new."

It looks that way, but the developmental history doesn't stop here: invasive growth and metastasis can come next (progressions, in Foulds' terminology), and these new properties also have nothing to do with loss of growth regulation directly. They are again new tricks which the cell learns.

Unfortunately, we must stop. Wouldn't it be possible to write out an arrest warrant for a tumor cell? Maybe with the following identification marks:
1. Increased cell division.
2. Simplified metabolic pattern (dedifferentiation).
3. Asocial behavior.

You can try, but with such a warrant you would make some very unpleasant discoveries; many a normal cell would be arrested, many a tumor cell would be overlooked:

1. Many tumor cells do divide faster than their surroundings, but this is not absolutely necessary. Many tumor cells simply forget to die, and in this way, too, the mass of a tissue is elevated above normal. Many therapeutic measures are intended to hit cells with high rates of DNA synthesis specifically. When the cells are not dividing more rapidly, these attempts, to put it mildly, have their problems: in this way much therapy is barking up the wrong tree.

2. If we exclude "differentiated" cells from the search, then the minimal deviation hepatomas and many other differentiated tumors remain unmolested. Finally,

3. "Innocent" lymphocytes that have floated out of the bone marrow would have to be scored as tumor cells because of their asocial behavior.

Just the few examples are convincing enough. None of these criteria alone is all that reasonable.

The situation is reminiscent of the Cheshire cat in *Alice in Wonderland*. You remember Alice's remark: "I've often seen a cat without a grin, but never a grin without a cat."

Everyone who tries to find the "pure clarity" of a definition in actual reality gets into a similarly confusing situation. So many aspects of a cancer cell (increased cell division, dedifferentiation, etc.) disappear upon closer examination, that finally there is nothing but a grin to remind us that cancer cells do exist, even if we can't define them clearly.

Doesn't that sound a bit too pessimistic — and without any really good reason? Why shouldn't cancer cells also be a "pluralistic society," each for a different reason having carved its niche out of different regulating fields and further developing to a considerable extent in its own fashion?

Exactly, and in this sense a pluralistic tumor theory would not be merely expedient, but the adequate description of reality.

SUMMARY: A PROGRAM FOR A COMPUTER

We still have to draw a balance, even if it comes off poorly. Of the many tumor theories, practically nothing remains that we can hold on to. There is still no satisfactory answer to the question, what is a tumor cell. One thing we can be sure of: cancer can be experimentally induced by the most varying means. But now as ever it is unknown whether there is a common denominator for all these different causes of cancer.

In the last 20 years, an almost incomprehensible mountain of facts has built up, but it is becoming more and more difficult to separate the important from the unimportant. Maybe a computer would help to separate the wheat from the chaff, and perhaps an electronic brain will someday forge the only possible tumor theory from the countless isolated findings. It might still be too early for that, but one could try formulating the problem for a computer. We will have to leave that to the mathematicians, but as a conclusion, permit us to dare the game of sketching examples for the induction and fate of the tumor cell in the manner of a computer program (Figure 51).

APPENDIX: MORPHOLOGICAL GLOSSARY

All **cells,** the basic building blocks of plants and animals, are constructed according to the same basic scheme (see Figure 21). *"Omnis cellula e cellula"* was Virchow's formulation, meaning that a cell can originate only from a mother cell.

Tissues are collections of many specialized cells. They are frequently divided into the two broad classes "connective and supportive tissue" and epithelial tissue. This division makes sense not only because of function, but because of developmental background: the "connective and supportive tissues" are derived from the middle germ layer **(mesoderm),** while the inner and outer germ layers **(endo-** and **ectoderm)** give rise to all of the epithelial organs and the nervous system. Generally, cells with specific assignments, such as nerve cells, are further distinguished from those that support them in their function, connect them, provide for their nourishment, etc.

Epithelia line or cover all of the inner and outer surfaces of an organism (epidermis, gastrointestinal mucosa, air passages, etc.). They are thus a "protective skin" against the environment and consequently

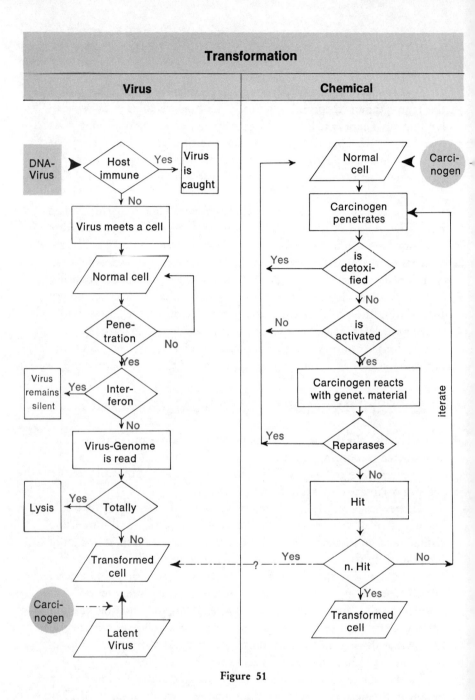

Figure 51

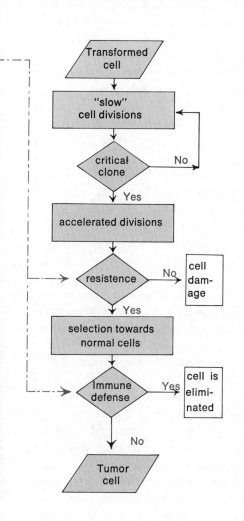
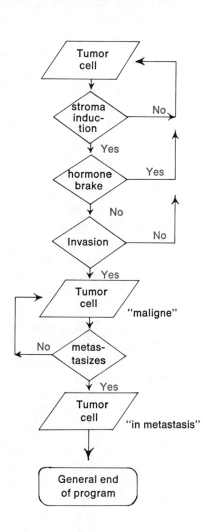

Figure 51 cont.

provide protective structures on the one hand (scales, hair, mucous); on the other hand, they have the ability to compensate for cell loss from special "basal cell layers" (see the role of the basal cells in hyperplasia on page 262). Distinctions are made among squamous epithelium cylindrical epithelium, and other variations according to cell form and aggregation. The "parenchymal" organs such as the liver, salivary glands, or mammary glands are also constructed from epithelial cells. These are stable tissues (see reparative regeneration, page 261).

The so-called **connective and supportive tissues,** totaling about 70–80 percent of the mass of higher animals, include bones, cartilage, fatty tissue, muscles, ligaments, tendons, etc. They hold the organism together. The connective tissue provides a superstructure and basis for epithelial tissue even in the smallest regions of tissue, and in this way helps to form the parenchymal organs.

Histology. Tissue can be observed under the microscope only after special pretreatment. In the routine procedures usual today they are first fixed in formalin or alcohol — made stable with sufficient preservation of structure — and imbedded in paraffin. The razor blades used in the early days have since been replaced by microtomes, with which remarkably thin slices are cut from the paraffin blocks. After being placed on a glass slide and stained with different dyes (hematoxylin and eosin), these slices can then be evaluated under magnification. It is striking that the DNA-rich nuclei read much more strongly with basic dyes (basophilic), while the cytoplasm preferably takes up acid dyes.

Histological **tumor diagnosis** draws conclusions primarily from the total picture of a tissue. It takes account not only of the cells of the tissue in themselves, but also judges them with respect to their exact arrangement in the tissue organization. Special attention is paid to the border between tumor tissue and normal tissue. "Architectural changes" stand in the foreground, then; the appearance of a single cell is not at all sufficient to identify it as a tumor cell.

Even so, many tumor cells are revealed by characteristic changes. **Exfoliative cytology** depends on this, using for instance cells taken from the uterus ("Pap smear"), or cells coughed up from the air passages. In a large cell spectrum, numerous "suspicious" signs can be determined which can be valuable within the framework of a search for indications of cancer.

Cells of **malignant tumors** represent an extremely heterogeneous population in contrast to the cell spectrum from normal tissue. Small and large cells are found next to each other, sometimes with large nuclei, sometimes with small, one staining strongly, one weakly (polymorphism, atypical population). The relationship between cytoplasm and nuclear mass has shifted in favor of the nucleus. Because of its high RNA level, the cytoplasm is more strongly basophilic than comparable normal cells. Visible signs of steady growth are the numerous mitoses that mostly do not proceed normally but precipitately. These pathological mitoses are recognized by chromosome sticking, breaks, or dispersal. Many times one gets the strong impression that division into two cells is not enough, since third and fourth divisions can be observed besides the usual mitoses. There is no longer an attention to exact distribution of genetic material, and the chromosome numbers in the individual cells of a tumor occasionally fluctuate widely (polyploidy).

Normal or **physiological regulation** of tissues shows that new cell formation is not a privilege of tumors. On the contrary, epidermal flaking is replaced from below daily; new blood cells constantly migrate into the bloodstream to replace overaged cells. Tissues that are constantly renewing themselves possess a type of cell entrusted with the production of offspring, so-called germ cells. In the skin these are the basal cells, and the stem cells in the bone marrow are partly responsible for the blood. They supply specialized (differentiated) functional cells to the same extent as they are consumed. Such exchange tissues can easily repair defects.

Reparative regeneration is a more difficult process in the so-called stable tissues, such as the parenchymal organs that have no germ cell layer. As far as they are able to, they must cover their losses from their complement of already specialized cells. A part of the cells have to "reverse poles", back from the functional state to mitosis. This permits restitution of the original tissue mass, making the "Prometheus story" possible.

Tissue metaplasia. If flat epithelial cells (such as in the skin) suddenly begin to grow from the "germ layer" of a cylindrical epithelium, or if simple connective tissue cells begin to produce bone at an inappropriate spot, this is called metaplasia. Such connective tissue cells have simply not yet "forgotten" to make bone, and "germ cells" of a cylindrical epithelium still "know" how to produce flat epithelium. They can't escape their own shadows, however. Epithelial cells never turn into connective tissue cells in metaplasia, and vice versa. Epithelial metaplasia usually has its origin in chronic damage (inflammation, mechanical irritation, etc.) and can thus be considered to be the result of misdirected regeneration. The developmental pathway of many malignant tumors (bronchial carcinoma, for instance) is only conceivable as passing over epithelial metaplasia: squamous (flat) epithelial carcinoma does not always have to have arisen from squamous epithelium.

NORMAL   8h   24 h   72 h

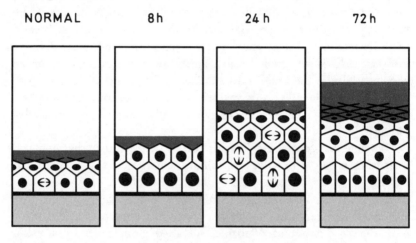

HYPERPLASIA OF MOUSE EPIDERMIS

Figure 52

Now if a regeneration process, in an epithelium for instance, follows the right track but overshoots the mark, **hyperplasia** results. Here new cell formation numerically exceeds the original cell complement. Let's look at the case of mouse epidermis (Figure 52). Normally the basal cells, the germ cell layer, rest on the basal membrane. The specialized (differentiated) cells are derived from these and in turn lead to the horny layer. (For our purposes we can ignore peripheral skin structures such as hair follicles, sebaceous glands, etc.) If this "interfollicular" epidermis is momentarily damaged with a suitable chemical "stimulant," hyperplasia results. First the epidermal cells swell (8 hours), and suddenly many more cells form from the basal cells than are sloughed off (24 hours). On a short term basis even cells of the higher layers (not only basal cells) can divide. Extensive horny layer formation follows this precipitate new synthesis (72 hours) and is later sloughed off. Now cell loss exceeds new cell production, and

10–12 days later the skin reaches its original cell level and gains the upper hand over the short-term interference with regulation. This example shows clearly that one can't talk about a tumor every time drastic cell replication takes place.

A long-term excessive hormonal stimulus can also lead to hyperplasia. The increased secretion of adrenal stimulating hormone by the pituitary results not only in increased production of adrenal cortical hormones, but also causes the cortex so to increase its cell complement as to meet the higher requirement for hormone production (hyperplasia of the adrenal cortex). This tissue replication is to be considered as an "appropriate response to changed hormonal correlations." The "cellular desired value" is reset at a higher level, and the number of normal cells is increased. If epithelial tissue either as cover tissue or in parenchymal organs exceeds a critical mass, there then result **papillomas** or **adenomas**, respectively.

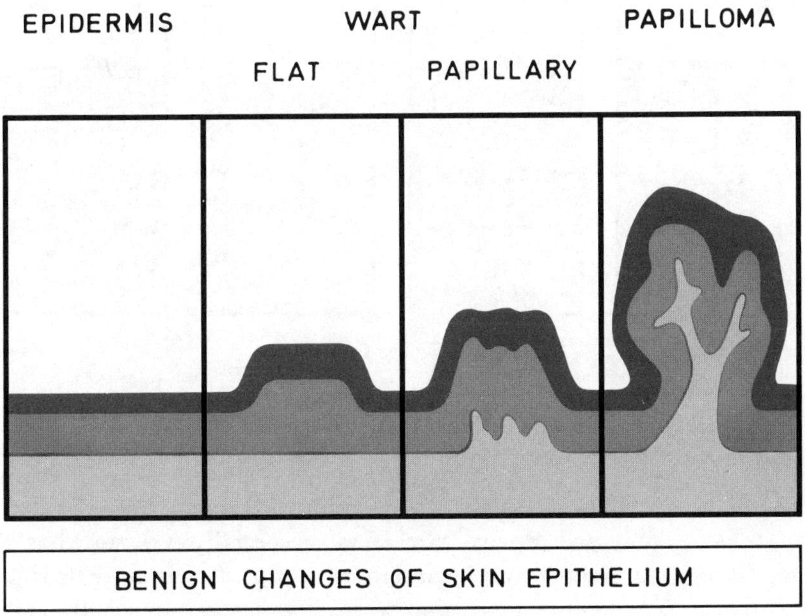

EPIDERMIS   WART   PAPILLOMA

       FLAT   PAPILLARY

BENIGN CHANGES OF SKIN EPITHELIUM

Figure 53

The epithelial cells have no more room on their connective tissue support, and to satisfy their supply requirements the nourishing "vascular-connective tissue" is forced to multiply along with them. The flat epidermal wart (Figure 53) can still be viewed as epidermal hyperplasia. In the papillary warts, the connective tissue support is no longer sufficient; it grows along with the epithelium outward, and in the papilloma finally reaches its greatest surface. Papillomas are already relatively independent "peripheral skin structures" with a certain autonomy. They can regress, however. If they are removed, they do not always have to reappear. If they are designated tumors, then they are spoken of as benign tumors. The corresponding multiplication of glandular epithelial cells is called an adenoma. Since adenomas lie "within" tissue, they simply appear as "tissue nodules." These are also benign tumors. The line separating these growths from malignancy is possibly most clearly seen from a presentation of a "carcinoma start."

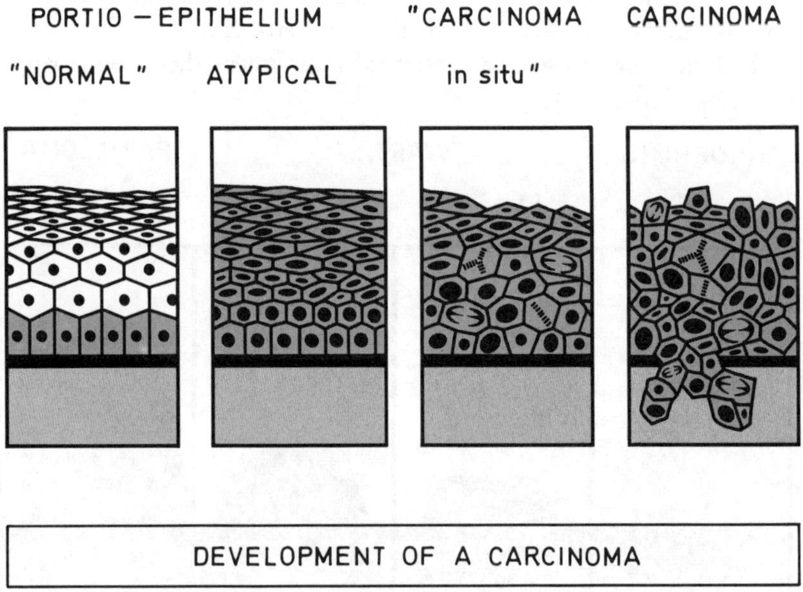

PORTIO — EPITHELIUM   "CARCINOMA   CARCINOMA

"NORMAL"   ATYPICAL   in situ"

DEVELOPMENT OF A CARCINOMA

Figure 54

The beginning of cervical carcinoma is especially well suited as a model of a "carcinoma start" (**carcinoma in situ**). At the outer uterine cervix, atypical epithelium can arise from apparently normally epithelium, which can be followed by a carcinoma in situ and finally a carcinoma, a cancer (Figure 54). In the first alteration, the "bright" cells ("normal" in the figure) are replaced by much more basophilic cells, i. e., darker staining ("atypical" in the figure). The nuclei chiefly of the basally located cells no longer have a regular size, but are polymorphous; the cell layering becomes less clear and finally disappears completely ("carcinoma in situ" in the figure). The irregular epithelium is characterized by increased cell multiplication and heavy staining of the nuclei and cytoplasm; to this are added unclear cell borders, pronounced nuclear polymorphism, shifting of the nuclear-cytoplasmic relation in favor of the nucleus, and numerous, occasionally atypical mitoses. As a whole, it is the picture of a malignant tumor. The "cellular army," however, is still at order arms on the border of its peaceful neighbor, hence "in situ". Only when the line of demarcation, the basal membrane is crossed and the cells grow invasively ("carcinoma" in the figure), do we speak of cancer, for now the atypical cells reveal their malignant, aggressive character, and only then do they metastasize. Logically, then, "carcinoma in situ" is really a spreading spot of mold.

Now we can delineate the concepts **"benign-malignant"** more precisely. The following table records the distinctions between benign and malignant tumors. This table may be valuable for tumor diagnosis, but has little to say about prognosis. A histologically benign papilloma of the trachea can rapidly stop breathing and kill the host. A "benign" brain tumor concedes a deadly risk for its host within itself. Conversely, a "malignant" skin carcinoma is relatively easy to treat and consequently not as dangerous (Table 7).

Table 7: Characteristics of Neoplasms

Benign	Malignant
Mostly slow growth	Frequently rapid growth
Grows expansively only	Also grows destructively and by infiltration
consequently	
Sharply delineated (no invasion, destruction, or metastases)	Poorly definable, growth into blood vessels, Metastasis
Architecture of the parent tissue largely retained (mature, differentiated tissue)	Severe deviation from the structure of the parent tissue possible, even so far as to be unrecognizable (Atypism and polymorphism in the tissue, cells, and cell nuclei)
Few mitoses	Mostly many mitoses

Carcinoma-sarcoma. Two groups of tumors are distinguished according to the two large classes of tissue. Epithelial tissues produce carcinomas, all "connective and supportive" sarcomas. Although connective and supportive tissue in man exceed epithelial tissue in mass by almost fivefold, carcinomas arise eleven times more frequently than sarcomas. Thus, from comparable tissue masses, about 50 times as many carcinomas as sarcomas appear. The frequency of carcinomas increases with increasing age, while the sarcoma rate remains about the same at all age levels. This is generally explained with the idea that the covering epithelia of the inner and outer surfaces are constantly the first to be exposed to summating carcinogenic stimuli.

Table 8: Nomenclature of Neoplastic Growth

Tissue of origin	Benign	Malignant
Epithelial tissue		
Skin	Papilloma	Skin *carcinoma*
Glands	Adenoma	Adeno*carcinoma*
Liver	Liver cell adenoma	Hepato*carcinoma* (hepatoma)
Pigment cells	Nevus	Malignant melanoma
Nerve cells	Glanglioneuroma	Neuroblastoma (only in young people)
Connective and supportive tissue		
Connective tissue	Fibroma	Fibro*sarcoma*
Cartilage	Chondroma	Chondro*sarcoma*
Bone	Osteoma	Osteogenic *sarcoma*
Muscle	Myoma	Myo*sarcoma*

The above table is intended to give only a small cross-section of the tumor spectrum and simultaneously show some examples of tumor nomenclature. From each tissue not only one tumor form but a whole spectrum of benign and malignant tumors can arise. In principle, only those tissues with cells capable of division should be able to produce tumors. Since nerve cells for instance no longer divide in adults, but do divide in children, correspondingly malignant "nerve cell" tumors are found only in young people (neuroblastoma, as an example). A few benign tumors from the above table are already known to us (Table 8).

Leukemias. If the tissues of origin of the white blood cells suffer a neoplastic change, they produce very large quantities of leukocytes — tumor leukocytes — and float them mostly out into the blood stream. This excess of leukocytes gives the blood a whitish appearance which suggested to Virchow the name white blood-leukemia. The principle forms of normal white blood cells derive from two sources: granulocytes from the bone marrow, lymphocytes from lymphatic tissue. Correspondingly, we have myeloid and lymphatic leukemias. In acute myeloid leukemia, even precursors of the granulocytes are released as tumor cells (Table 9).

Table 9: Classification of Leukemias

Cell type	Origin	Leukemia	"Solid" tumor form
Granulocytes	Bone marrow	Acute and chronic myeloid leukemia	Myelosarcoma
Lymphocytes	Lymphatic tissue	Chronic lymphatic leukemia	Varying lymphomas, lymphosarcomas

If routing of the cells into the blood stream does not occur, then we speak of an aleukemic leukemia, and the tumorous growth character of the disease is its distinguishing characteristic, since the cells pile up where they are produced. This extremely simplified table gives only an overview. The tumorous nature of lymphatic leukemias is mostly underscored by visibly enlarged lymph nodes. In the myeloid form, the normal blood-forming bone marrow is displaced by "tumor marrow," resulting in a deficiency of red blood cells (anemia) and normal granulocytes. This can result in a high susceptibility of the host to infection. Leukemia cells cannot cope with bacterial invasion because of their functional inferiority.

Ascites tumors. Another "liquid" tumor form is known, primarily from experimental cancer research. Occasionally, ascites tumors can be prepared by injecting tumor material into the peritoneal cavity of experimental animals. The tumor cells then induce the formation of ascites fluid in which they are individually suspended, nourish themselves, and multiply like true one-celled organisms. They relinquish supporting connective tissue or a vascular supply. The recipient animal is practically degraded to a living nutrient medium. Many such tumor lines have already been maintained for several decades through hundreds of passages. This is a practical demonstration of the "immortality" of these tumor cells which, similar to tissue culture cells, obviously do not "age" as normal cells do (**Transplantation tumors,** see page 127).

The **growth** of **malignant tumors** (in solid neoplasms) is primarily characterized by invasion and destruction of neighboring tissue and by resettling of metastases. Many phenomena are blamed for **invasive growth** and are covered in more detail on pp. 89 ff. These are increases of the negative charge on the surfaces of tumor cells, their increased, absolutely ameboid mobility, and their cohesion. Membrane alterations that lead to loss of contact inhibition and an increased internal pressure within the tumor are also considered to be responsible.

Lytic enzymes of the tumor tissue are also blamed for **destruction** of normal tissue. If a **primary tumor,** i. e., a neoplastic growth at its place of origin, remains attached to its parent tissue and its surroundings, and if it were to grow invasively and destructing only, it would still be possible to remove it and return the situation a long way toward a healthy condition. A malignant tumor becomes extremely dangerous only through **metastasis,** the settling of tumor cells in distant organs via the blood and lymph streams; in other words, by a generalization of the disease. The migrating tumor cells can attach to capillary walls, multiply, and grow into a new tumor, metastasis, or **secondary tumor,** with all the properties of the primary tumor. The relationship is occasionally so obvious that primary tumors are not infrequently recognized by their metastates. A lung metastasis consisting of hepatoma cells immediately proves the existence of a liver cell carcinoma, even if the latter is latent. A detailed treatment of metastasis is found on pages 74 ff.

Autoradiography. The objection is repeatedly lodged against histology that it concerns itself only with fixed, that is dead material — with artificial products. Autoradiography meets this objection to a certain degree. Max Beckmann quoted a Cabalist once: "If you want to comprehend the invisible, you must delve as deeply as you can into the visible." For the microscopist, "invisible" would mean: infer processes and causal connections from momentary exposures of histological preparations. Here autoradiography goes a decisive step further, by making events "directly" visible ("dynamic microscopy"). Autoradiography makes use of the ability of radioactive material to blacken photograph emulsions. If we offer a tritium (^{3}H)-labeled building block for nucleic acid or protein to a cell, this labeled compound is taken up and incorporated regardless of its radioactivity (Figure 55). If after fixing the preparation, we then layer over a sensitive photographic emulsion or a film, we can then observe under a microscope (after exposure and development) small black dots in the film directly above those places where the cells incorporated labeled material. Of course this assumes that the labeled end product in the cell is not lost during preparation and that all of the unused building blocks can be extracted. Using this "criminalistic" method, it is possible to trace individual labeled molecules in the cell, since these molecules reveal themselves.

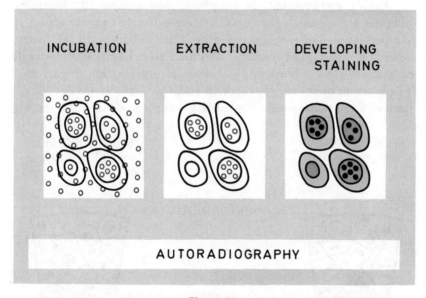

Figure 55

Here is an example: if we offer a labeled specific DNA building block to a culture of only identical cells for a short time (pulse labeling), then in a certain percentage of the cells removed shortly thereafter we observe a blackening of the film above the nuclei. Only these cells have used DNA building blocks during the period of the experiment, and only these cells have newly synthesized DNA (Figure 51). One is looking at what the cells are "doing."

Tumor stroma. Solid tumors do not consist only of tumor cells, but also dispose of connective tissue which gives them their structural support, and naturally blood vessels to take care of metabolic requirements. Connective tissue and vascular system, collectively called stroma, derive from the respective surroundings of the tumor. The tumor presses the normal tissue into this form of serfdom. Osteoblastic metastases demonstrate these facts, where carcinoma cells compel the local bone cells to prepare a bony skeleton for them. Stroma in many carcinomas even goes so far that the connective tissue components predominate over the tumor cells, leading to the characterization of scirrhous (hard). In their destructive work, tumors often do not stop even at their own stroma and thus cut the life lines for large areas of their own structure, leading rapidly to large necroses in areas that usually already have deficient vascularization.

Tumor construction. In neoplastic nodes, especially in transplanted tumors, the highest proliferative activity is mostly found at the periphery. The frequency of mitosis decreases toward the center, where the oldest, most "mature" cells are found. Horny squamous cell carcinomas clearly show this geographical organization (Figure 56). In the center of the smallest growth nodes we come across "pearling" derived from mature cells. An entirely comparable picture is possible

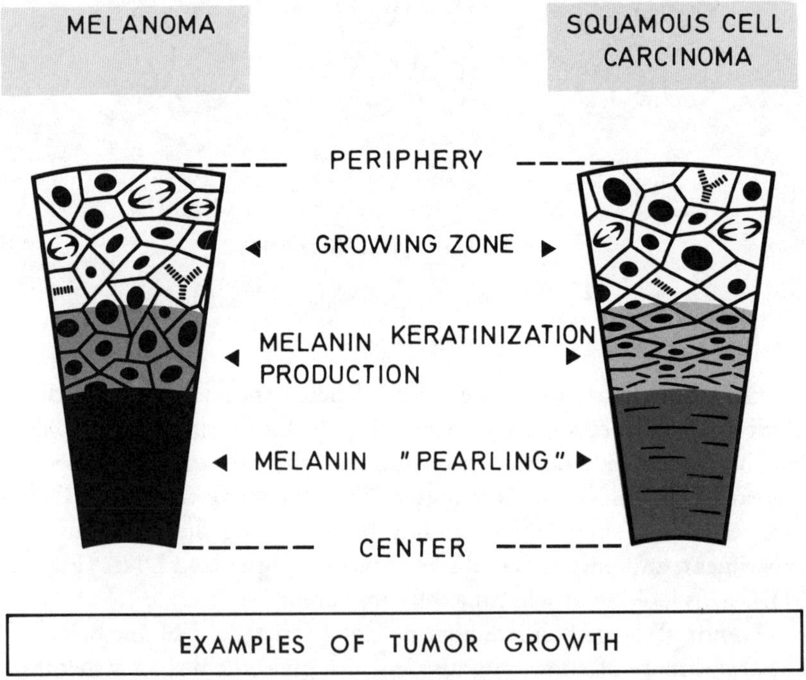

EXAMPLES OF TUMOR GROWTH

Figure 56

in malignant melanoma (Figure 56). With a mitosis rate decreasing toward the center, the cells unpigmented until then suddenly recall their capabilities and begin to produce their differentiation product, melanin. They lose their ability to divide and die off into a deep black necrosis.

The pair of concepts **differentiated and dedifferentiated** describes how far tumor cells deviate from the degree of specialization (degree of differentiation) assumed by their normal parent cells (matrix) within the organism. The degree of differentiation of a tumor cell is determined from its most mature representative, such as the "pearls" or the melanin-producing cells. Frequently, a microscope is not even needed. If mammary gland tumors produce milk, or tumors of the adrenal cortex flood the male rat with so much hormone that changes in habits even to feminization are observed, this is sufficient proof that tumor cells can still be functionally intact. Tumor cells that divide in especially rapid rhythm do not have any time to display their specialties and produce differentiation products such as horn, melanin, milk, or hormones. They are dedifferentiated. And the fact that dedifferentiated tumor cells are especially malignant because of their faster multiplication is immediately obvious. This can even go so far in transplanted tumors, that what were originally carcinomas completely turn into sarcomas.

The **degree of malignancy** in the "life of a tumor" does not have to remain constant either. It can change, and usually increases. Following short-term remissions after radiation therapy or chemotherapy, especially fast-growing resistant tumor cells may be selected, which occasionally bring about the death of the host very rapidly. They have become more "virulent." Thus, a "hands-off" policy is even a therapeutical necessity for many forms of tumors in certain phases of the disease. This is immediately reminiscent of the therapy resistance of many bacterial infections, especially staph. Ascites tumors in experimental animals are especially malignant or virulent. With the consequent transplantation of Yoshida sarcoma cells from rat to rat, it has been possible to so reduce the cell count necessary for fatal "infection," that it is now possible to kill a rat with only a single one of these cells.

The comparison with an infection is also brought up because many ascites tumors grow not only in their species of origin but also in other species and kill the new hosts. Thus, somatic cells have become parasites, and only the means of transport is lacking (still dependent on the experimenter's syringe) to give rise to a new infectious disease. A mosquito could enter the picture here, an *Anopheles ascitica*, which would propagate these tumor cells. A hamster sarcoma has in fact been transferred with the aid of a mosquito *(Aedes aegyptii)*. In this instance it had only been necessary to pen up the normal animals with the mosquitos and the tumor-bearing animals (Figure 57). The mosquito had completely replaced the hypodermic syringe (Banfield). The obvious objection, that tumor viruses and not tumor cells were transferred, could be easily answered: if male hosts were penned up with female hamsters and mosquitos, the females developed tumors which had the male karyotype. If a virus had induced a tumor only after entering the females, these tumors would have had to show a female karyotype.

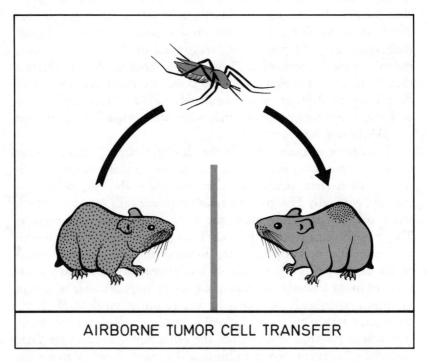

AIRBORNE TUMOR CELL TRANSFER

Figure 57

The cancer cell can, therefore, in the truest sense of the word, tread the path back from a multicellular organism to a parasitic unicellular organism. Whether this is to be considered as the height of degeneration or as regeneration depends strictly on one's perspective.

REFERENCE WORKS

Direct quotations were taken from the following:

Allison, A. *Europ. J. Cancer.* **3**: 481 (1967/68).

Ambrose, E. *In* The Biology of Cancer. (E. J. Ambrose and F. J. C. Roe, eds.) London, 1966.

von Ardenne, M. Die selektive Verstärkung einer primären Krebszellen-schädigung als Fundamentalprozeß der Krebs-Mehrschritt-Therapie. Turin lecture, 1969.

Bauer, K. H. Das Krebsproblem. Berlin, 1963.

—, and Ott, G. Materia Medica Nordmark. Uetersen, 1965.

Beijerinck, M. W., citet by G. Williams. *Virus Hunters.* New York, 1960.

Berenblum, I. Cancer Research Today. Oxford, 1967.

Bierwisch, M., cited by G. Schiwy. Der französische Strukturalismus. Hamburg, 1969.

Braun, A. C. *Scientific American.* **213,** Nov. (1965).

Bullough, W. S. The Evolution of Differentiation. London, 1967.

Burnet, F. M. *Science.* **133**: 307 (1961).

Dulbecco, R. *Scientific American.* **216**: April (1967).

Druckrey, H. *In* Potential Carcinogenic Hazards from Drugs. R. Truhaut, ed. Berlin, 1967.

Fletcher, C. M. Krebs-Dokumentation und Statistik. G. Wagner, ed. Stuttgart, 1966.

Foulds, L. *Cancer Res.* **14**: 327 (1954).

— cited by J. Leighton (which see, below).

— Neoplastic Development. Vol. 1, London, 1969.

Gaylord, H. R., cited by E. D. Day. *Ann. Rev. Biochem.* **1962,** 549.

Habel, K. *Cancer Res.* **28**: 1825 (1968).

Hallion, cited by C. Oberling (which see, below).

van Helmont, J. B., cited by W. Osler. The Evolution of Modern Medicine. New Haven, 1921.

Henschen, F. *Gann* **59**: 447 (1968).

Hieger, I. Carcinogenesis. London, 1961.

Huxley, J. Biological Aspects of Cancer. New York, 1960.

Kant, I. Metaphysische Anfangsgründe der Naturwissenschaft 1786. Cited by H. E. Fierz-David. Die Entwicklungsgeschichte der Chemie. Basel, 1952.

Kissen, D. M. Ann. New York Acad. Sci. 164: Art. 2 307 (1969).

Leighton, J. The Spread of Cancer. New York, 1967.

Lettré, H. *Universitas.* **21**: 49 (1966).

McKinnel, R. G., et al. *Science.* **165**: 394 (1969).

von Nagel, A. Fuchsin, Alizarin, Indigo, Ludwigshafen. (no date given)

Oberling, C. Krebs, das Rätsel seiner Entstehung. Hamburg, 1959.

Potter, V. R. *In* Molecular Basis of Neoplasia. M. D. Anderson Hospital, Austin, 1962.

Reid, E. Biochemical Approaches to Cancer. Oxford, 1965.

von Rezzori, G. Maghrebinische Geschichten. Hamburg, 1958.

Schmähl, D. Entstehung, Wachstum und Chemotherapie maligner Tumoren. Aulendorf, 1963.

—, C. Thomas and K. König. *Z. Krebsforsch.* **65**: 342 (1963).

Schopenhauer, A. Philosophische Menschenkunde. A. Bäumler, ed. Stuttgart, 1957.

Stewart, S. E. *Scientific American.* **203**: Nov. (1960).

Szent-Györgyi, A. Bioelectronics. New York, 1968.

Taylor, G. R. The Doomsday Book. London, 1970.

Thompson, d'Arcy W. On Growth and Form. J. T. Bonner, ed. Cambridge, 1961.

Warburg, O. Molekulare Biologie des Malignen Wachstums. H. Holzer and A. W. Holldorf, eds. 1966.

— *Naturwissenschaften.* **42**: 30 (1955).

Wightman, W. P. D. The Growth of Scientific Ideas. New Haven, 1951.

Zilber, L. A. *J. Nat. Cancer Inst.* **26**: 1311 (1961).

Data from the following works were used for tables and illustrations:

Ambrose, E. J. See above. (Figure 22).

Anders, F. *Experientia.* **23**: 1 (1967). (Figures 43, 44, 45).

Bauer, K. H., and Ott, G. Materia Medica Nordmark. Uetersen, 1965.

Benjamin, T. L. *J. Mol. Biol.* **16**: 359 (1966). (Figure 42).

Boyland, E. Aktuelle Probleme aus dem Gebiet der Cancerologie II. H. Lettré and G. Wagner, eds. Heidelberg, 1968.

Bryan, W. R., and M. B. Shimkin. *J. Nat. Cancer Inst.* **3**: 503 (1943). (Figure 9).

Daudel, P., and R. Daudel. Chemical Carcinogenesis and Molecular Biology. New York, 1966. (Figure 8; Tables 1, 2).

Druckrey, H. See above. (Figures 10, 11; Tables 3, 4).

Holley, R. W., and J. A. Kiernan, *Proc. Nat. Acad. Sci. USA* **60**: 300 (1968). (Figure 27).

Horne, R. W. *Scientific American.* **208**: Jan. (1963). (Figure 38).

Robertson, J. D. *Scientific American.* **206**: April (1962). (Figure 25).

Schramm, G. *In* Molekularbiologie. T. Wieland and G. Pfleiderer, eds. Frankfurt, 1967. (Figure 38).

Wagner, G. Grundlagen der Tumorgenese. Ludwigshafen, 1968.

Warburg, O. See above. (Figure 29).

For additional reading

The Biology of Cancer. Edited by E. J. Ambrose and F. J. C. Roe. London, 1966.

The Cancer Problem. By A. C. Braun. New York, 1969. The author is a developmental biologist who has spend his life studying plant tumors.

Neoplastic Development. By F. Foulds. London, 1969. Only Vol. 1 of a planned series has appeared so far.

Das Krebsproblem. By K. H. Bauer. Berlin, 1963. This work makes the connection between experiment and clinical practice.

Chemical Carcinogenesis. By D. B. Clayson. Boston, 1962. Although 10 years old, this book has not been equaled in its balance between coverage of a broad field and critical evaluation of experiments.

Review articles on more limited areas can be found in the following series:
   Advances in Cancer Research, New York.
   Methods in Cancer Research, New York.
   Progress in Experimental Tumor Research, Basel.
   Recent Results in Cancer Research, Berlin.
   UICC-Monograph Series, Berlin.

INDEX